The Crisis of Care

The Crisis of Care

Affirming and Restoring
Caring Practices in the
Helping Professions

EDITED BY

Susan S. Phillips and Patricia Benner

GEORGETOWN UNIVERSITY PRESS / WASHINGTON, D.C.

Georgetown University Press, Washington, D.C. 20057
© 1994 by Georgetown University Press. All rights reserved.
Printed in the United States of America.
10 9 8 7 6 5 4 3 2   1994
THIS VOLUME IS PRINTED ON ACID-FREE OFFSET BOOKPAPER.

This work was funded in part by the Lilly Endowment, Inc.

Library of Congress Cataloging-in-Publication Data

The Crisis of care : affirming and restoring caring practices in the
   helping professions / Susan S. Phillips, Patricia Benner, [editors].
        p.   cm.
      1. Caring.   2. Helping behavior.   3. Professional ethics.
   I. Phillips, Susan S.   II. Benner, Patricia E.   III. Title: Helping
   professions.
   BJ1475.C75   1994
   174--dc20
   ISBN 0-87840-558-5
                                                    94-9702

Contents

Preface

This book argues that examining our exemplary caring relationships can prompt us to redesign the structures and processes of our public caregiving institutions in order to better facilitate practices of caring. The premise is that we must first understand the best of our caring practices by attending to the notions of the good life and skilled ethical comportment embedded in them. Listening to narratives of practice enables that kind of attention, and the reader will find many narratives in this book, both free-standing and incorporated in chapters.

There is a subtext in each chapter that concerns recovering a vision, concrete strategies, and moral space for caring practices. Teaching, nursing, medicine, psychotherapy, and pastoral ministry are written of from the inside in terms of excellent practice and qualitative distinctions (Kierkegaard, 1962; Rubin, 1984; Taylor, 1989) that interact with it in the everyday work of helping professionals.

The authors in this book write of actual, less than ideal, circumstances and the real people who practice care within those circumstances. If caring practices are to be noticed, affirmed, and restored, this must happen in the context in which they take place. The reader is invited to examine the narratives in terms of the practices of care illustrated in them. How is the story itself constituted by ethical concerns? What is being protected? What are the visions and relational issues of the one caring and the one cared for? In what ways are technological, managerial views of the person overcome so that the other person is encountered as a particular person with a distinct history and concerns? We believe it is essential to recover the vision of what is possible in actual practices today in order to discover the mandates for reshaping our institutional structures, environments, and economics to serve attentive, sustaining, and healing relationships.

We have a strong tradition of considering theory liberating and practice enslaving or unenlightened; however, this is not always the case (Taylor, 1989). As the narratives in this book show, excellent, instructive practice that embodies distinctions of worth creates the vision of what ought to be and how to live toward that vision. A dominant strategy in all the helping professions has been to objectify and standardize as much of the professional activity as possible in the quest for quality control. But this strategy obscures the requisite judgment and particularized relationships required in the helping professions.

A helping professional is not a teacher, nurse, physician, psychotherapist, or pastor simply by virtue of possessing large quantities of information and adhering to objectifiable codes of behavior that limit (or exclude) judgment and response (Rubin, 1984). These practitioners *do* possess the necessary information and behavior codes; they also have experientially embedded standards and visions of excellence. They have notions of what counts as excellent and poor practice, qualitative distinctions about what counts as preserving personhood, fostering growth, restoring wholeness and integrity, offering encouragement, and so on. By examining concrete instances of caring practice we can recover distinctions of worth within the practice.

There are many paradoxes in caring practices. If the helping professional acts on general principles to "act caringly" as a means of self-improvement or salvation, or as a means of controlling fears of finitude and vulnerability, then the caring practice will suffer. The one cared for will be objectified, enslaved, or infantilized rather than liberated and strengthened by care. These are real dangers that have fueled the epidemic level discourse on pathologies of care, burnout, and codependency. The parallel danger is to pathologize care in general for fear of inauthentic care or from failure to hope that authentic, nonparasitical care is possible and essential even in a world where it seems—and is—impossible ever to care adequately for all needs. A huge burden on individuals accompanies the North American view that caring is psychological, a private attitude possessed by certain persons. We no longer understand our connection, however tenuous, with moral sources and communities of care and, so, see ourselves as stoically shouldering the concerns and labor on our own.

In the best caring practices both the community and the individual serve and are preserved. In narratives of excellent practice there is an ethical discourse of learning that goes both in the direction of the one caring and that of the one cared for. Caring relationships set up the possibility of mutual realization, not a power discourse in which one person gives, helps, and does not learn from the other, while the other person merely receives and learns. The reader will see in the narratives many instances in which the caregiver learns and is transformed by the caregiving relationship. Such encounters teach much about our shared humanity and the spiritual dimensions of assisting fellow human beings in the midst of suffering, loss, and living the finite gift of life. Those receiving care are called upon to trust and appropriate the help that is offered. That, too, requires attentiveness, attunement, learning, and the relinquishing of obstructive control for the sake of care.

In our culture of independence and self-determination, the practices of opening oneself to another's care are even more emaciated than those of giving it. As Robert Wuthnow points out in *Acts of Compassion* (1991, p. 175; see Bellah's discussion of this in his chapter), we are people who remember Jesus' story of the Good Samaritan in "its subjective, individual, and moralistic aspects." We identify ourselves with the hero whom we see as acting outside of a community of care. We do not like to think of ourselves lying helplessly by the side of the road. However, we all do rely on the kindness of strangers and others, and the restoration of caring practices involves recognizing what it is to enter relationships of care that undermine radical independence and self-determination.

We, the editors, have learned much from the authors of this book and from those who have become part of the community of conversation around this project. Because much of the material in this book comes from personal experience and heartfelt commitments, we have been moved by the trust of those writing on these pages.

This book grew out of conversations among many people at New College Berkeley, a small graduate school for the laity, affiliated with the Graduate Theological Union in Berkeley, California. Since the late 1970s New College Berkeley has been a locus of study and dialogue for scholars and helping professionals interested in reflecting on everyday life and practice in the light of faith. The courses sponsored by NCB have displayed a breadth and depth of interest and reflection mirrored in this book. NCB courses have been a place where personal narratives have been considered rich sources of knowledge, both metaphysical and ethical. We trust that this book will be useful for courses and discussions where the goal is to examine the everyday challenges of living out an ethic of care.

The editors of this book met through New College Berkeley seminars and community gatherings while we were both graduate students at the University of California, Berkeley. At NCB we found a community in which to explore the spiritual and moral dimensions of our scholarly work. While our professional lives have diverged during the past years, we have sustained these conversations through friendship and through NCB.

We express our gratitude to the New College Berkeley community of scholars that has supported and shaped this work in numerous ways; specifically, to Richard Benner, Joel Green, Frank and Lois Andersen, David Gill, Bill and Grace Dyrness, Laurel and Ward Gasque, David Batstone, Margaret Alter, and many others. While an explicitly Christian institution, we have experienced New College Berkeley as a school and community with sufficient faith to open conversations wide and allow wisdom and goodness to enter through many channels.

We also must acknowledge the teaching and writing of Robert Bellah, Hubert L. Dreyfus, Jane Rubin, and Charles Taylor who have supported this work with their ideas and their encouragement. For intellectual challenges and financial support we are indebted to James Wind and the Lilly Endowment Inc. Much gratitude is due John Samples of Georgetown University Press who understood the significance of this work for ethics and public policy.

There are others who have enabled us in this work and deserve mention here. Maryann Aberg, David Anderson, Mima Baird, Robert Bevier, Charles Eaton, Sharon Gallagher, Bill Ghirardelli, Carrie Ghirardelli, Suzanne Gordon, Kim Hamilton, Abby Heydman, Bill Jersey, Bonnie Johnston, Sister Mary Brian Keller, Amy Keltner, Jeff Lazarus, Victoria Leonard, Leonard Nielson, Ellen Ogle, Earl Palmer, Kate Peterson, Carole Rudy, Harriet Smith, Josephine Wood Smith, Lee SmithBattle, David Soister, Don Strongman, Mary Thompson, Janet Visick, and others helped us think about a conversation among the helping professions and encouraged us when the work seemed daunting.

Bill Visick was a special friend and source of encouragement during the shaping of this book. He cared for us and taught us about faith, hope, and love. Throughout the three years of work on this book we have been held by the love of family: Susan's parents and brother, David, Elizabeth, and Dave Sanders, Patricia's sister June Hagman our husbands, Steve Phillips and Richard Benner and our children, Andrew and Peter Phillips, and John and Lindsay Benner. They have given us the love that makes care possible.

SUSAN S. PHILLIPS

PATRICIA BENNER

REFERENCES

Kierkegaard, Soren, *The Present Age* (New York: Harper and Row, [1846] 1962).

Rubin, Jane, *Too Much of Nothing: Modern Culture, the Self and Salvation in Kierkegaard's Thought* (Unpublished doctoral diss., University of California, Berkeley, 1984).

Taylor, Charles, *Sources of the Self: The Making of the Modern Identity* (Cambridge, MA: Harvard University Press, 1989).

Wuthnow, Robert, *Acts of Compassion: Caring for Others and Helping Ourselves* (Princeton, NJ: Princeton University Press, 1991).

Introduction

SUSAN S. PHILLIPS

> If the world has not approached its end, it has reached a major watershed in history equal in importance to the turn from the Middle Ages to the Renaissance. It will demand from us a spiritual blaze; we shall have to rise to a new height of vision, to a new level of life, where our physical nature will not be crushed, as in the Middle Ages, but even more importantly, our spiritual being will not be trampled upon, as in the Modern Era.
> —Alexsandr Solzhenitsyn,
> *A World Split Apart*

There is a crisis in caring for persons that cuts across the boundaries of the helping professions. Patients in hospitals feel depersonalized and processed, students suffer from inadequate attention, clients wonder if therapists really care about them, and parishioners feel unknown in their places of worship. Caregivers are rewarded for efficiency, technical skill, and measurable results, while their concern, attentiveness, and human engagement go unnoticed within their professional organizations and institutions.

The manifestations of our failure to care satisfactorily for people are legion. Social indexes indicate that the gap between the rich and poor is widening. The unemployment rate rises, and workers receive fewer employee benefits. This country has one of the least adequate family support systems in the Western world. Violence is increasing, and the prison population grows without reform. Though the United States is a wealthy country, its medical care statistics are as alarming as those of developing nations. Our public school system is crumbling, and people are searching for alternatives.

The failure to care for our citizens undermines the best efforts of science, technology, and management. Much of the burden of this fail-

1

ure falls on caregiving professionals who stand in the breach between the policymakers of our society and our own outstretched hands. Many caregiving professionals experience a conflict between the vocation to care for persons and the industry of caring for manageable parts and aspects of human beings.

CARE IN A CONTEXT OF IMPERILED PERSONHOOD

Increasingly in the helping professions, personhood and caring have been eclipsed by the depersonalizing procedures of justice distribution, technological problem-solving, and the techniques and relations of the marketplace. These strategies are attempts to solve the distortions that came with earlier visions of care, such as sentimentality, pity-blame equations, and the disenfranchising of persons. Our modern strategies suffer from their own pathologies that also create victims and adversaries: In the middle of the night a bleeding man arrives at the emergency room of a hospital, and questions about his insurance precede any inquiries about his physical condition; a young couple join a church and immediately find themselves approached as potential "giving units"; a high school student finds no one to help her get the classes she needs in order to apply for the advanced training she needs to pursue her vocation.

The objectification of persons within the relationship of caregiving leaves many caregivers frustrated, confused, and ashamed of their genuinely compelled caring while many receivers of care are humiliated, angry, and alienated. Our culture has omitted a significant dimension of human being from consideration and attention. Iris Murdoch writes, "The charm and power of technology and the authority of a 'scientific outlook' conceal the speed with which the idea of the responsible moral spiritual individual is being diminished" (1992, p. 426).

From Max Weber onward, social observers have lamented the loss of the soul in modern society. The soul, while elusive of definition, has to do with the embodied, socially constituted, vulnerable and resilient, free yet dependent, earthly and transcendent nature of human beings. Elements of modern society marginalize and damage the soul by their failure to deal with that which is irreducibly complex and fraught with paradox. In our efforts to simplify, codify, categorize, control, explain, and diagnose, we fail to understand and care for each other. Instead of meeting obligations to free and restore the human soul, we seek the power to manipulate. As dependable servants of a growing democracy, we place our faith in rationality, procedural justice, technology, efficiency, productivity, and profitability. Ethically significant capacities and practices, like those that allow us to care and respond to care, have been eclipsed. In order to develop systems that process the masses fairly, we have lost touch with the fact that our abstract systems depend on qualities of persons and relationships that elude quantification and codification. These qualities deserve respect, even reverence; the systems we construct to help us order the world cannot survive without the soul breathing life into them.

Many have claimed that the modern age is characterized by a loss of meaning and sanctity, in which "qualitative distinctions are weakened by gnawing reflection" (Kierkegaard, [1846] 1962, p. 43; Taylor, 1989). Caring practices, in which distinctions having to do with qualitative worth always are embedded, are banalized and diminished by the privileging of bureaucratic systems of processing people. We seek contracts and tested techniques to fend off the anxiety and risk that come from reliance on socially complex and meaning-laden human practices. We avoid involvement and commitment for fear of loss and disappointment as well as the nobler fear of potential injustices. We reflect on others from an analytical stance that protects us from knowing them as persons while enabling us to process them as cases, clients, and ciphers. It is dangerous for helping professionals to believe that others populate the kind of existential landscape called a "wasteland" by Eugene Peterson (in his chapter "Teach Us to Care and Not to Care").

The kind of reflection that discounts people's hopes, understandings of goodness, and distinctions of worth is deadening and, potentially, deadly. Detached simplification in the service of manipulation is an effective strategy with inanimate objects; it is both ineffective and ethically unacceptable for encountering what is animate and endowed with meaning. Albert Borgmann writes:

> [T]he dominant discourse about the future of our society is composed of the vocables of prognoses, projections, extrapolations, scenarios, models, programs, stimulations, and incentives. It is as though we had taken ourselves out of reality and had left only objectified and disavowed versions of ourselves in the universe we are trying to understand and shape. We vacate our

first-person place and presence in the world just when we mean
to take responsibility for its destiny. . . .

We live in self-imposed exile from communal conversation
and action. The public square is naked. American politics has
lost its soul. The republic has become procedural, and we have
become unencumbered selves. (1992, pp. 2–3)

This is, according to Borgmann, the crisis of modernity.

In unencumbering ourselves, we have shed much of our humanity. In our emphasis on legal ethics and rights, we have failed to meet
our moral obligations of compassion and goodness. As we head
toward a new millennium, people attuned to our social failures are
beginning to question the faith we have placed in "the dominant discourse." We have fallen short of the democratic ends we sought to
achieve with procedural justice, technology, and strategic planning,
and there is a creeping despair as we consider the monumental challenges of repairing our public institutions.

Our move toward rationalizing the relations between people
was neither accidental nor malevolent. In part it was guided by ethical promptings to limit the effects of prejudice, special interests, entrenched power structures, and various forms of elitism. Countless
people have been protected by a strict adherence to principles of freedom and rights ensured by those who would not otherwise respond
to them with compassion and sympathy. Marginalized groups found
footholds in the developing structure of procedural rights and ethics
and benefited from a system that thwarted the dominance of self-
interest and exploitation. However, the demand on us now is to re-
animate our principled systems and find respectful and just ways to
recognize the values, hopes, commitments, and practices that will restore our schools, neighborhoods, health centers, and places of worship (see Taylor, 1992). Taylor, Borgmann, and others are calling us to
leave our armchairs, step outside the laboratory, take off our gloves,
look beyond manuals of codes and procedure, and involve our en-
cumbered selves.

Without minimizing the significance of our achievements, a nation
of pragmatic individualists is awakening to the consequences of inat-
tention to the young, the old, the disabled, the sick, and the poor who
represent the conditions of our shared humanity and vulnerabilities.
The approach of managing situations and fixing problems has failed to
nurture robust communities that promote well-being. Speaking of the

crumbling of Communist regimes under the revolt of the human spirit, Vaclav Havel, poet and leader of Czechoslovakia, said: "Man's attitude to the world must be radically changed. We have to abandon the belief that the world is merely a puzzle to be solved, a machine with instructions for use waiting to be discovered, a body of information to be fed into a computer in the hope that, sooner or later, it will spit out a universal solution" (1992). Similarly, Robert Bellah and his co-authors in *The Good Society* (1991, p. 274) claim that in the United States "we have settled for easy measures that have distracted us from what needs to be attended to and cared for."

RESTORING AND NURTURING OUR PRACTICES OF CARE

Clearly, the challenge facing us is widespread and profound. It requires the courage to pay attention to complicated problems that cannot be solved mechanically or easily. By our social philosophers and our fellow citizens we are being called to introduce into ethical consideration aspects of human life that have to do with imagination, meaning, caring, and what is good, and to do so without eroding the necessary checks we have placed on our self-serving proclivities.

Many believe that in the last century our public faith was broader; that, in addition to the rational underpinnings of our society, there were practices of faith, community, and celebration as well as the remnants of craftsmanship and regard for responsibility, civility, courtesy, and care. The helping professions saw themselves as bearers of our collective faith. "Helping" and "caring" were not suspect. The relationship between religious faith and work was captured by concepts like vocation, charity, service, and care. The errors of care were different than those made by "unencumbered selves," yet they, too, created victims and adversaries. Paternalism, the manipulation of others masquerading under the guise of helping and caring, and caregiving motivated by guilt and shame are a risk when work is seen as a meaningful "calling" rather than a job. However, stripping relations of significance is only one radical and risky way of guarding against the ravages of personal insecurity and ambition.

Today the cultural pendulum has swung away from finding spiritual or moral significance in caring service, and we question the moral sources as well as the project of caring for others. We have become cynical about the possibility of goodness. We question why one person cares for another. Is it healthy? Is it to satisfy the caregiver's emotional needs for power, love, or fulfillment? Those who shape institutions and policy have attempted to correct the errors of the helping professions by substituting economic and bureaucratic controls for the practical wisdom and moral intents of caregivers. Feminists, aware of the gender stratification that consigns women to subordinate caring functions, wonder whether we can salvage an ethic of care from the structures of oppression. Critics of religion, similarly, ask if doctrines of submission and self-sacrifice are weapons against spirit and equality. These cautions are important, and ethicists of care must be careful of trafficking in idealistic illusions about care. But we dare not abandon care in a retreat into cynicism and indifference.

In a world of inequality, difference, uncertainty, and power politics our social practices must be undergirded by a net of impartiality created by quantitative standards, market controls, and rationalizable entitlements. This net is essential; however, we have lost our commitment to and language for that which suspends this net. The compelling force and recognition of "what needs to be attended to and cared for" (Bellah et al.) must suspend the safety net undergirding our practices of care. Weaving and maintaining the net is insufficient; we must hang it on something.

The multiple moral sources, habits, virtues, skills, and practices that animate our liberal democracy are capable of suspending this net of democratic rights, justice, and suitable technique, but they have been vitiated and hidden in order to protect the mechanisms of impartiality. They have been excluded from recognition and from the public square. The mechanisms of impartiality, therefore, lose their animating connection with visions of the good life and commitments to the freedom and dignity of the individual. While a culture's visions and commitments can be protected by procedures of justice, these procedures are not sufficient for creating senses "of the good, the holy, the admirable" (Taylor, 1992, p. 72). Those are lodged in our everyday private and public lives, in the traditions, communities, practices, and relationships that enable us to know what deserves attention and is worthy.

Having fled the dangers of partiality and the distortions of care, we have run into the dangers of depersonalization and disengagement, into a wasteland disconnected from the wellsprings of our souls. Though we commit ourselves to fairness and reason, we are persons who care and who care about some things more than others. We understand ourselves in terms of our sense of what matters, or, in

Charles Taylor's words, "against a background of 'strong evaluation.'" Taylor describes personhood as follows:

> [T]o be a full human agent, to be a person or a self in the ordi-
> nary meaning, is to exist in a space defined by distinctions of
> worth. A self is a being for whom certain questions of categoric
> value have arisen, and received at least partial answers. Perhaps
> these have been given authoritatively by the culture more than
> they have been elaborated in the deliberation of the person con-
> cerned, but they are his in the sense that they are incorporated
> into his self-understanding, in some degree and fashion. My
> claim is that this is not just a contingent fact about human
> agents, but is essential to what we would understand and recog-
> nize as full, normal human agency. (1985, p. 3)

Given this understanding of a person as constituted by what is cared
for and as living in a world of distinctions of worth, the attempt to
leave such considerations out of human relationships seems futile at
best. This dimension of human agency cannot be eradicated; it only
can be ignored, or recognized.

Questions of significance and goodness matter to people. Everyday life reveals that to us, though in certain settings we may try to
anesthetize ourselves to deeper meanings and moral reactions. Such
numbing mutes despair, pain, and outrage, but it also tranquilizes us
against what can make life good, rich, and joyous. When we mute our
evaluative capacities, we deprive ourselves of helpful information
about ourselves and others, and we lose the opportunity of learning
from the qualitative distinctions others make. Martha Nussbaum
writes, "Trusting the guidance of a friend and allowing one's feelings
to be engaged with that other person's life and choices, one learns to
see aspects of the world that one had previously missed" (1990, p. 44).
She makes the same claim for literature as she does for friendship as
nurturing knowledge, and the same claim is being made, here, for
relationships of caregiving.

A portion of the culture's ethical discourse about meaning and
goodness takes place indirectly in art and literature, while, for the
most part, it is excluded from professional and public debate. When
surfacing our distinctions of worth in our public conversation, we
must strive to cultivate the discourse within the safeguards of the
web of impartiality and justice. To do otherwise would open us to the

errors of intolerance, fanaticism, injustice, and tyranny. The use of any religious or secular tradition as a means of exclusion and devaluation of the freedom and traditions of others violates our ability to hear and see one another. The risk is one of entering a dogmatism, narrowness, and unholy self-righteousness that is destructive. The authors of this book share a faith that the restoration and affirmation of human goods embedded in caring practices does not have to lead to destruction, while the suppression of those goods will.

In the helping professions, both ethically and practically, the provision of good care cannot be sustained solely by decisions about who has a right to what. An adversarial system of rights discourses exclusive of regard for meaning, concerns, and the practical knowledge embedded in practices not only blinds us conceptually, practically it yields an insufficient environment for the flourishing of patients, students, clients, and others in need of care. The child does not have a right to level eye contact from a teacher, yet the child feels cared for by and may learn more from the teacher who comes close to help shape a letter. The patient has no right to an encouraging touch on the hand or a telephone call at home two weeks after the office visit, but both acts might promote healing. A church member has no right to a pastoral visit during which the pastor prepares a meal, but that act of care might be life-changing.

A care system based on rights alone sterilizes professions still referred to as "helping" and "caring." It cultivates polarity rather than engagement. The honoring of rights and fulfilling of legal and professional obligations are essential to caregiving, but they are the safety net, not the skillful artistry that is itself that which warrants the net's protection. To overlook the caring practices, concerns, and "strong evaluations" of the caregiver is to miss what is significant.

Within the different caring professions dialogues emerge and submerge about what the relationship ought to be between the professional and the person requiring care. Some argue for a scientific and procedurally just stance that might protect both the caregiver and the receiver of care from the complicated and possibly stressful effects of interpersonal emotional involvements. Others argue for the motivation, direction, and meaning that are derivative of personal concerns, caring, and commitment. The helping professionals and scholars contributing to this book are on the side of acknowledging meanings, concerns, commitments, inclinations, intuitions, and fallibility. They are aware of the difficulties and risks involved in this approach, but believe the risks are greater when the fullness of human nature is denied.

Practices of caring are shaped by engagement with others and learning with others what is helpful and good; therefore, practices contain ethical and practical knowledge. In this book the reader will encounter practices from several helping professions. The practices shed light on one another as we are able to see common and different understandings of competing goods, ethical concerns, and moral sources dwelling within the practices. The ethical and spiritual illumination possible from practices of care may contribute to the redemptive "blaze" called for by Solzhenitsyn. To be redemptive the blaze must be one of illumination from practice rather than an immolation based on "right" belief.

SEEING PRACTICES FROM WITHIN THE EXPERIENCE AND MEANING OF PERSONS

The contributors to this book link their caring practices to the sources of their understandings, not only of rights and standards within their particular professions, but also of other dimensions involved in living a good life and attending to what matters. For many of the contributors, understandings about the value of persons and the nature of interpersonal relationships derive from personal faith that is both a path and a gift. In an age when we hear much about "empty" selves, and suspicion of care, the authors of this book hope for the affirmation and restoration of caring practices for the sake of finite, spirited persons.

The vitality of caregiving lies in the practices of giving care, yet the articulation of what occurs is not easy, even for those engaged in the practices. This book brings multiple perspectives to bear on the crisis of care and caring practices that survive despite all. The narratives in this book demonstrate quality of care and openness to care. The relationship of giving and receiving care is nonrationalizable and is best understood when seen fully and in context. To dissect it into components, stages, or systems is to lose significance, just as the study of a dead or even a caged bird gives a pallid, unnatural, and incomplete understanding of a bird. The narrative enables us to see what takes place and to grasp significance as it emerges.

The incorporation of narratives in this book is integral to its nature and purpose. Drawing on the tradition of biblical exegesis and interpretive phenomenology, this editor is most influenced by the teaching and writing of Patricia Benner (*From Novice to Expert* and with Judith Wrubel *The Primacy of Caring*), as well as by the many published works of Robert Coles (on the lives of children and *The Call of Stories: Teaching and the Moral Imagination*); the work of James McClendon (*Ethics: Systematic Theology, 1*); and the works of Stanley Hauerwas (*Naming the Silences* and *Why Narrative?*) and those of Alasdair MacIntyre (especially *After Virtue*). The reader is invited to dwell with the story and enter into dialogue with it. H. Richard Niebuhr writes of two ways of hearing a narrative:

> Events may be regarded from the outside by a non-participating observer; then they belong to the history of things. They may be apprehended from within as items in the destiny of persons and communities; then they belong to a life-time and must be interpreted in a context of persons with their resolutions and devotions. ([1941] in Hauerwas and Jones, 1989, p. 31)

The narratives presented here belong to "the destiny of persons and communities" (Niebuhr), and readers should approach them as "'participators in a fond attention'" (Nussbaum, *Ibid.*).

To engage with a narrative requires a leap of faith that suspends disbelief in order that what is told can be heard. Response to a narrative is not unlike a caregiver's response to the one cared for, for listening to a story requires us to involve ourselves in another's world of time, embodiment, relationship, meaning, and concern. Patricia Benner writes, "To be told a story is almost to become a participant in it" (1991, p. 29). In forming a story the teller has made choices about what is important to tell. The reader of the story has the opportunity to enter the storyteller's world.

The narrators in this book offer their experiential learning about caring, impediments to caring, failures to care, and the capacities inherent in responding to care, as well as their fears, hopes, and concerns about good caring. What is told and what is left unsaid in a narrative reveal significance and insignificance and what is considered good. Caring practices require a community and are seldom stories of heroic, independent acts. Care is relational, creating more than we expect and at other times showing us the limits of "helping."

The chapters in this book are written by practitioners and theorists. The authors are widely known and regarded as experts in their fields. Each has taken a position for the importance of practice and the caring skills and relationships within practice. Each has spoken out against the objectification and commodification of persons and practices that mark contemporary helping professions. Voices from medicine, nursing, teaching, ministry, sociology, theology, and philosophy join together in articulating a vision for caring practices. The voices are distinct and capable of disagreement; they originate in differing life situations and cultures. However, they call us to a vision of personhood and the possibility of goodness that can be discovered in the caring practices of the helping professions.

Practitioners and scholars come together in this book because their understandings of caring impact one another. Though this approach seldom has been used in a book about the helping professions or one about the ethic of care, many have argued for conversations among practitioners and scholars. Taking an interpretive stance, we understand the human sciences as informed by the lives, meanings, ideas, experiences, and knowledge of people they seek to know. More specifically, any social scientific knowledge of practice must submit itself to the lived knowledge of practitioners and enter into dialogue with those practitioners.

In turn, practitioners are shaped by the curricula of their professional schools, the thinking of scholars of practice, and the culture of their professions which is affected by popular theoretical work in the field. Scholars within the systematic disciplines are, as Craig Dykstra argues, ". . . essential for helping communities and persons know what they are doing and why as they engage in these practices. They are also essential for the continuing criticism and reform of these practices, the goods internal to them, and the knowledge that they make possible" (in Wheeler and Farley, 1991, p. 56).

The scholars represented in this book have a deep reverence for the knowledge of practice and do not view theory as a higher realm of knowledge. They seek to avoid the objectivist stance of viewing the social world as a "spectacle" and seek the knowledge possible through "practical relation to the world, the preoccupied, active presence in the world through which the world imposes its presence, with its urgencies, its things to be done and said, things made to be said, which directly govern words and deeds without ever unfolding as a spectacle" (Bourdieu, 1990, p. 52).

The authors also do not use theology as an epistemological trump card over faithfully lived practice. It is likely they would agree with Rabbi Leib about the Torah: "'A man should see to it that all his actions are a Torah and that he himself becomes so entirely a Torah that one can learn from his habits and his motions and his motionless clinging to God'" (Buber, 1947, p. 66). The following is a Christian articulation of the same point:

> Theology, modern or classical, can also be an excuse, an alibi, and permit us to get swamped in a rarefied world of insights and concepts where real life cannot bubble up any more. "Are you a theologian?" asked a hermit of Mount Athos of a monk from the West who had introduced himself as such. "Ah, a saint is a real flower. But compared with a saint a theologian is only an artificial flower. It imitates a flower's rich display of colour but spreads no fragrance, and bears no fruit." (Louf, 1992, pp. 17–18)

The reader is invited to learn from the habits, motions, stillness, fragrance, and fruit of the practices of caring that are shown in these pages. They offer a full-blooded and rich knowledge, unlike that of the arid, observational knowledge we often encounter in scholarly books.

The sort of knowledge that caring practices (and other practices) make possible is context-dependent, historically developed, and concerned with action as well as deliberation. Aristotle, writing of *phronesis* or "practical wisdom," describes such knowledge as a "reasoned and true state of capacity to act with regard to human goods" (1973, Book 6: 1140b:20). Such knowledge, unlike physical science, is concerned with things particular rather than universal, with things variable, and with "things human and things about which it is possible to deliberate" (Aristotle, 1141b:7). Practical wisdom is a knowledge embodied in persons and communities. People experience themselves as being solicited, called, pushed, thrown, and drawn by their concerns and their situations into particular actions that cannot be replicated cybernetically based on principles, energies, and strategies. The chapters that follow employ narrative, interpretation, and deliberation in an attempt at a *phronesis*-based consideration of caregiving in the helping professions.

CHAPTER SUMMARIES

Sociologist Robert Bellah in "Understanding Caring in Contemporary America" calls for paying attention to what constitutes a good life. In a time when even the private domains of life (the "lifeworld") are being colonized by market concerns and by strategies of control and profit-maximization, Bellah argues for a rich, interpersonal world of people attending to one another and the quality of life, for the cultivation of institutions that encourage attentiveness, and for governments that sponsor the caring efforts of communities and institutions. From a stance of faith and hope, Professor Bellah beseeches Americans to listen and see, to adopt an ethic of responsibility, attentiveness, care, and moral discourse rather than the paradigm of control and commodification.

In "Caring as a Way of Knowing," Patricia Benner presents notions of the good life and knowledge embedded in the expert caring practices of nurses. Care is explored as creating possibilities and salience, as well as practices that allow human beings to show up as human, interdependent, worthy, and requiring care. Patricia Benner examines various nursing practices as ways of knowing and caring for the patient. She advocates such practical knowledge as essential to a health care system dominated by technological and economical views of health and care.

Drawing on T. S. Eliot's poem *Ash Wednesday,* in "Teach Us to Care and Not to Care" pastor Eugene Peterson addresses the complexities of distinguishing between authentic caring and control masquerading as care. Dr. Peterson claims that the place in which caring occurs is sacred, and that even ministers get distracted from the sacred and lured to the bustling life of selling wares and promoting doctrines. In entering the sacred realm in which caring takes place, we must be humble and willing to wait for understanding. The knowledge of how to care, the practical wisdom of it, must emerge within the situation. The beginning is adoration, receptivity, and hope. If we approach the world as if it were a wasteland to us, we fail to find meaning and possibility in it; we end up acting like minor providences shoring up a derelict god or exhausted resources trying to manage other supplies.

Pediatrician E. Dawn Swaby-Ellis, in "The Caring Physician: Balancing the Three Es—Effectiveness, Efficiency, and Empathy," provides examples of the multiple demands on the physician's role and examines the moral sources for the character of the physician. Professor Swaby-Ellis shares her own religious and familial moral sources for caring and demonstrates these in narratives from practice, thus allowing us to see how strong evaluations shape her caregiving practices.

Master teacher Jaime Escalante is committed to "Preparing Students for the World." In his chapter by that title, he writes of his sometimes questioned, widely admired, and always intense teaching of poor minority students for whom education is the primary vehicle for transporting them out of poverty and marginality. Like the surgeon who oversteps standards of practice in order to save lives, so Mr. Escalante provokes our ethical sensibilities as he goes to extremes to save the lives of his students. In this chapter, the understanding of the lives and situations of the students is essential to evaluating the way Mr. Escalante navigates through a tension-ridden field of competing ethical goods. The reader can ask, What sort of world does he invite his students to enter?

In "The Corrosion of Care in the Context of School," educator Anna Richert states that "At the core of teaching practice that would help kids grow . . . is care." However, schools are particularly hard hit by the "crisis of care" affecting our society. Professor Richert tells of the increasing challenges and dangers teachers face as they attempt, with care, to teach students in settings of urban chaos. She considers ways to promote pedagogical caring and attempts to answer the twin questions: How can we establish a school culture based on an ethic of care—a school culture that provides care for both students and teachers? And, finally, how can we not?

Ethicist David C. Thomasma contrasts "technological fixes" with the more difficult processes of human engagement in "Beyond the Ethics of Rightness: The Role of Compassion in Moral Responsibility." Because technology empowers individuals beyond their normal capacities, it challenges the bounds of temperance and wisdom. Medical paternalism is fueled by technological powers that cause physicians to believe that they know what is best for the other. Rationalistic approaches to bioethics that focus on what is the right thing to do rather than compassionate attentiveness to the particular person, context, and human concerns cannot adequately defend against technical and medical paternalism. Without naively discounting technology, Thomasma proposes compassionate contextualism as an alternative to rationalistic ethical decision-making. An ethic of compassion is based upon human connectedness, and the full human experience of suffering that humanizes both the sick and the healthy.

In "Caring as Gift and Goal: Biblical and Theological Reflections," biblical scholar Joel Green examines New Testament moral sources for caregiving practices. The Bible describes a relationship between the Creator and human beings that constitutes an ethic of care and responsibility that transcends, but does not negate, an ethic of justice and obligation. Persons and communities are called to ethical comportment shaped by visions of what is good, by God's character, and, for Christians, by the life and person of Jesus. This ethical comportment is marked by servanthood, not by manipulation and domination; by foot-washing, feeding, and dwelling amongst, rather than by practices of brain-washing, manipulating, and lording over.

Philosopher Charles Taylor, in "Philosophical Reflections on Caring Practices," provides a powerful and succinct statement of the current debates about forming a pluralistic society that responds to more than market forces. Written in response to the rest of the chapters and narratives in this book, Professor Taylor's chapter is a critique on moral philosophy that focuses only on acts and not on ways of being with and responding to others. In terms of creating a society capable of valuing caregiving that is molded by concerns, Professor Taylor argues that we must learn to feel and appreciate the force of moral sources that we do not share in order to build a society where we can form coalitions around visions of the good life.

This book explores the multiple faces of caregiving through stories of care, the reflections of caregiving practitioners, and the interpretation and contextualizing of caregiving within a larger social and theoretical framework by scholars. The three kinds of approaches mingle within some chapters as well as throughout the book as a whole.

REFERENCES

Aristotle, *Nichomachean Ethics*, in *Introduction to Aristotle*, ed. Richard McKeon (Chicago: The University of Chicago Press, 1973).

Bellah, Robert N., Richard Madsen, William M. Sullivan, Ann Swidler, and Steven M. Tipton, *The Good Society* (New York: Alfred A. Knopf, 1991).

Benner, Patricia, *From Novice to Expert: Excellence and Power in Clinical Nursing Practice* (Menlo Park, CA: Addison-Wesley, 1984).

Benner, Patricia, "The Power of Our Stories," *Radix*. 20 (3), Fall, 1991.

Benner, Patricia and Judith Wrubel, *The Primacy of Caring: Stress and Coping in Health and Illness* (Menlo Park, CA: Addison-Wesley, 1989).

Borgmann, Albert, *Crossing the Post-Modern Divide* (Chicago and London: University of Chicago Press, 1992).

Bourdieu, Pierre, *The Logic of Practice*, trans. Richard Nice (Stanford: Stanford University Press, 1990).

Buber, Martin, *Ten Rungs: Hasidic Sayings* (New York: Schocken Books, 1947).

Coles, Robert, *The Call of Stories: Teaching and Moral Imagination* (Boston: Houghton Mifflin, 1989).

Dreyfus, Hubert L. and Jane Rubin, "Kierkegaard, Division II, and Later Heidegger." In Dreyfus, *Being-in-the-World: A Commentary on Heidegger's Being and Time, Division I* (Cambridge, MA: The MIT Press, 1991).

Dykstra, Craig, "Reconceiving Practice," in *Shifting Boundaries: Contextual Approaches to the Structure of Theological Education*, eds. Barbara G. Wheeler and Edward Farley (Louisville, KY: Westminster/John Knox Press, 1991).

Hauerwas, Stanley, *Naming the Silences: God, Medicine, and the Problem of Suffering* (Grand Rapids, MI: Eerdmans, 1990).

Hauerwas, Stanley and L. Gregory Jones, eds. *Why Narrative? Readings in Narrative Theology* (Grand Rapids, MI: Eerdmans, 1989).

Havel, Vaclav, Speech at the World Economic Forum, Davos, Switzerland, February 4, 1992.

Heidegger, Martin, *Being and Time*, trans. J. Macquarrie and E. Robinson (New York: Harper and Row, 1962).

Kierkegaard, Soren, *Fear and Trembling*, trans. Alastair Hannay (London: Penguin, [1843] 1985).

Kierkegaard, Soren, *The Present Age* (New York: Harper and Row, [1846] 1962).

Louf, André, *Tuning into Grace: The Quest for God* (Kalamazoo, MI: Cistercian Publications, 1992).

MacIntyre, Alasdair, *After Virtue* (Notre Dame, IN: Notre Dame University Press, 1981).

McClendon, James, *Ethics: Systematic Theology, 1* (Nashville, TN: Abingdon Press, 1986).

Murdoch, Iris, *Metaphysics As a Guide to Morals* (New York: Allen Lane, The Penguin Press, 1992).

Niebuhr, H. Richard, "The Story of Our Life," in *Why Narrative? Readings in Narrative Theology*, eds. Stanley Hauerwas and L. Gregory Jones (Grand Rapids, MI: Eerdmans, 1989).

Nussbaum, Martha, *Love's Knowledge: Essays on Philosophy and Literature* (New York: Oxford University Press, 1990).

Solzhenitsyn, Alexsandr, *A World Split Apart* (New York: Harper and Row, 1978).

Taylor, Charles, *Human Agency and Language: Philosophical Papers, 1*, (Cambridge: Cambridge University Press, 1985).

Taylor, Charles, *Multiculturalism and "The Politics of Recognition"* (Princeton: Princeton University Press, 1992).

Taylor, Charles, *Sources of the Self: The Making of Modern Identity* (Cambridge: Harvard University Press, 1989).

NARRATIVE:

When Life Threatens

HARVEY PESKIN

Love never moves and distresses us so much as when watching the children of abused parents try to heal their parents' pain by shouldering it
for them, even impossibly leeching it from them. I am not speaking
about those abused parents who, feeling themselves unlovable, exact
what is really a loveless loyalty from a son or daughter by abusing the
child even as they—the parents—had been abused in their own child-
hoods. Such faithlessness between generations changes the natural
bond of a child's relational trust into a fragile tissue. I am speaking of
abused parents who do not hurt their child as they had been hurt, and
who can still commit themselves and their offspring to an unbroken
connection of care. Such parents are often those who were betrayed
and traumatized, not in the primal relationship with their own parents,
but in the havoc of war or prison, or in the terror of genocidal annihilation. In my psychotherapeutic work, I know them as Holocaust survi-
vors and their children. This narrative describes a culminating moment
from my long-term psychotherapy with an adult child of Holocaust sur-
vivors that constituted a transformative crisis of caring for my patient,
her family, and for myself.

The therapeutic work leading to this moment is not out of the ordinary for a young adult: simply, a young woman's struggle to decide
whether to marry against the wishes of her parents. It was not her parents' rejection or ostracism that Helen worried about in marrying a non-
Jew. Through reworking the past in her therapy, Helen, mature and
reflective but emotionally subdued and cautious, had already become
aware that her fear of rejection had little real basis because her parents
were essentially approving and loving. This newer awareness was
shown, for example, in her recapturing a childhood memory that first
appeared as a fragment in which she was running home in wild desperation, starkly afraid of her mother's punishment for playing past supper-

time. Helen could not answer my question about what her mother actually did to her until some time later in our work when she recognized her own quite deep anxiety about her mother's war suffering. The rest of the memory of her mother's reaction to Helen's running home late came forward. Now she remembered that mother did not punish her, but had warmly soothed her and given her something to drink.

In such therapeutic work the patient became aware that her fears, now understood as out of all proportion to what really happened, masked anxieties that were set in motion by her sense that she had failed in her paramount duty not to aggravate the bitterness of her parents' Holocaust suffering. But such intense faithfulness also stopped Helen from crediting her parents with any essential capacity to live outside of their Holocaust suffering (as in her trouble remembering that her mother could take pleasure in soothing her as a young girl). So much had my patient been living with this sense of her parents' unalterable suffering that she identified her mission to relieve her parents' pain not with any enhancement of their satisfaction in living, but only with their avoidance of new pain. And if Helen could not imagine their capacity for joy, she also could not believe in her parents' capacity to enjoy their child's pleasure. So, in her memory of running home late for supper, Helen could not tell her mother that she was late because she was having a wonderful time competing with her friends around the school track.

The struggle to marry at all showed that Helen had taken that special step forward in personal growth when a tightly bonded daughter is ready to understand that separating from one's parents does not have to mean abandoning them. Considering marrying a non-Jew played into Helen's fear that she would betray her parents and fail forever in her mission to bring no more harm into their lives. She anguished over the stress of the marriage on her aging parents. Would marrying a non-Jew shorten their lives? Would her father's mild heart condition worsen? Would her mother's usual brooding become a fixed depression? Helen's own brooding virtually reached the point of standing accused by herself of siding with the Nazi persecutors who once pursued her parents' annihilation.

In the midst of this spiraling dilemma between love for parents and partner, Helen came to her weekly therapy with a resolute announcement of a way out: she and her lover were quite prepared to postpone marriage indefinitely, even, if need be, until after the death of her mother, the parent Helen felt would be devastated by the marriage.

Helen appealed to the exquisite airtight correctness of this plan that would hurt no one and protect her mother from this devastation. As a modern woman Helen believed that living together without a legal marriage was no hardship, certainly not compared to her mother's hardship if she did marry.

I was astonished and alarmed at hearing Helen's plan, to an extent that seemed out of all proportion to her tone of mature reasonableness. Her plan in any case was not an extraordinary one, especially in traditional households. Knowingly or not, many of us postpone all sorts of important life decisions—like making, leaving, or changing a job, a home, or a marriage—'til after the death of a loved one, most often a parent, whom we are afraid would otherwise be severely injured emotionally. Helen's long-term therapy had already helped her stop dismantling the good fortune of her life as she became aware that doing so could not rescue her parents from the abyss of the Holocaust. However, carrying out her plan for postponing marriage seemed for Helen stronger than the illumination of this major insight. Marriage was in an unassailable class of its own. Here, quite consciously, Helen seemed unwilling to give up the belief in the power of her guilt to heal her parents' pain.

In the same session, I said this to Helen: "Do you know that if you hold off marriage until your mother dies you'll find yourself wishing for her death?"

This is the culminating moment I was speaking about. I have often been drawn back to what was at work in myself, in Helen, and in our therapeutic relationship that led me to respond to her announcement with this grim prediction, a prediction that virtually precipitated the crisis that the patient sought to avoid. You probably know that therapists are warned against presuming foreknowledge of the patient's life (as in my prediction) because doing so tends to lead patients to believe they must change who they are into the image the therapist has for whom they should become in the future. Yet, in that moment of Helen's therapy, my well-trained uneasiness about intruding into a patient's future seemed like a nicety my sense of crisis could ill afford. I intended to be as steadfast as I knew how to shake her out of her stubborn indifference to how she was putting her future in peril.

The peril I suddenly envisioned was that, by devising a plan that would inevitably provoke death wishes, Helen was already sentencing, indeed dooming, herself to the ultimate self-punishment of making herself into her parents' murderer. My intervention was meant, therefore, to help her avoid being turned into a self-scorned person who henceforth would deserve nothing. Far from worrying about molding the patient in the therapist's own image, I was concerned with protecting Helen's own good and growing image of herself as one who cared deeply for her parents and felt their deep care for her. For me, the crisis of caring in this moment was how to take care of her before her doubt about the right to marry destroyed the relationship with her partner.

After this, the crisis passed quickly. Marriage did not belong in a separate class of its own after all, but was really the culminating step and test after many previous ones, tests by Helen of the parents and the therapist to be understood in the context of her lifelong wish to bring into harmony her personal autonomy and her deep relatedness to her parents. My grim words had not frightened her into submission so much as they reawakened a sense of being watched over by me and her parents. The crisis I triggered by my bleak prediction called up in myself a sense of therapeutic responsibility for a patient's future growth and development that I had not experienced so fully before. This experience, among others, has helped me to examine more critically the received professional wisdom of avoiding attention to the dimension of the future in the patient's life course.

The wedding took place with a fully alive and happy mother and father in attendance.

My emphasis has been on Helen's difficulty in confidently trusting her sense of being loved and cherished by her mother and father, although the deeper therapeutic work showed that she was loved and cherished. I believe it was not some hidden parental abuse that the therapy simply did not get to, but rather Helen, in her faithful mission of relieving her parents' suffering, carried not her own but *their* Holocaust experience of being uncared for and scorned.

In retrospect, I think the wording of my prediction to Helen of her impending self-punishment for postponing marriage was demanded by the need to stop the looming possibility that she could become their persecutor, no longer their loving child. That, I think, is the posthumous victory that Hitler would relish: Jew turned against Jew. This, the Jewish therapist could not allow. For the non-Jewish therapist, making such a dire prediction would be in the spirit of the Christian rescuer of Jews who boldly signaled to them the unseen danger ahead rather than remain, like too many others, a passive onlooker to their annihilation.

Understanding Caring in Contemporary America

ROBERT N. BELLAH

Almost two and a half years ago we heard a presidential inaugural address that called for "a kinder, gentler America." There is not much evidence that we are becoming kinder and gentler—indeed there is a good deal of evidence that we are becoming less so. Before addressing some of the cultural tendencies and the social practices that make kindness and the practices of caring increasingly difficult in our society, I want to say something about the semantics of "caring." The distinction needs to be drawn between caring as a sentimental psychological attitude and caring as a responsible practice, aware of its own limits.

Allan Bloom and other neo-conservatives have attacked the language of "care" and "caring" as part of the self-serving vocabulary of the new class, of which the helping professions form a significant part, that is, bleeding-heart liberals who like to see as many people as possible as victims. My own sense is that the neo-conservative attack on care and caring is itself cynical and contributes to the decline of caring practices. Yet, the neo-conservatives do have a point. Genuine caring is a practice based on moral commitments with which certain subjective feelings may or may not be associated, but it is not primarily a psychological orientation. Genuine caring does not see those in need primarily as victims. Genuine caring involves a profound sense of moral responsibility, but it does not imagine that caregivers have the technology or the power to heal all wounds and cure all ills. I will return to these issues.

Some of the following material is taken from *The Good Society* (Robert N. Bellah, Richard Madsen, William M. Sullivan, Ann Swidler, and Steven M. Tipton, NY: Random House, 1991).

The *cultural* tendencies that I see as endangering practices of caring seem to be located in a broad spectrum of American culture, especially middle-class culture. This tendency is expressed best in an ideology of radical individualism that my co-authors and I analyzed in *Habits of the Heart* (Berkeley and Los Angeles: University of California Press, 1985), but that I would like to illustrate with some examples from Robert Wuthnow's excellent book *Acts of Compassion* (Princeton University Press, 1991), which has the significant subtitle *Caring for Others and Helping Ourselves.*

One ameliorating tendency in our utilitarian society is the recognition that individuals do, after all, have feelings and that these feelings should be expressed, yet we must question in some instances how limited the range of feelings is that is being emphasized. One of the major motivations stressed by volunteer agencies that encourage people to give time and money to helping others is that such activity will "make you feel good." Wuthnow describes an advertisement for a well-known international relief agency recently carried in a Christian magazine with a large national circulation.

> At the top was the familiar face of a needy child, dark skinned, with large, sad eyes. Beside her picture in bold, black, underlined letters half an inch high was the word SPONSORSHIP. Below this, filling up nearly a quarter of the page in equally huge letters were the words "It'll Make You Feel Good." But in case the reader might have missed this message or not understood it, the ad contained more. Three times in quarter-inch bold section headings the message was repeated. "You'll Feel Good . . . knowing that you can help stop her hunger. You'll Feel Good . . . knowing that Jesus' love for children has been demonstrated through your compassion. You'll Feel Good . . . knowing that you're touching this hurting world." "Please become a sponsor today," it concluded: "You'll feel good about it." (p. 86)

Many volunteers recount that occasionally help at a soup kitchen or with Meals on Wheels "really makes them feel good," sometimes asserting that their volunteer activity is more for themselves than for the people they help. A volunteer fireman says, "I don't do this to help people. I do it to make myself feel good about helping people." Another of Wuthnow's subjects said, "If I stop to help somebody cross the street, I do that because I want to feel good. It gives me that feeling that I've done something good for the day." The same person ventured the opinion that selfishness and compassion "are really the same thing." One may wonder whether we should take such assertions at face value, since Americans seem almost ashamed to admit that they might do anything out of altruistic motives.

But the stress on "feeling good," as Wuthnow argues, may actually endanger the relatively high commitment to volunteerism in our society. He points out that when asked what makes them feel good, Americans usually rate quite a few activities higher than helping others and that a great deal of helping others involves hard, often painful work. It may involve what it has become almost taboo in America to mention, sacrifice. Indeed, Wuthnow found out something quite revealing about the meaning of sacrifice to Americans today. Forty-two percent of his national sample said that a major reason to be a kind and caring person is "I want to give of myself for the benefit of others"; but when in a subset of the sample Wuthnow changed the wording to "I want to sacrifice myself for the benefit of others," the percentage dropped from 42 to 15 percent. It is hard to imagine Jesus, as Wuthnow notes, saying to his disciples, "'Take up your cross and follow me—it'll make you feel good'" (p. 87), but some televangelist has probably already said as much.

The poignant reality of helping others is that it often does involve sacrifice and by no means always makes one feel good. Wuthnow quotes Albert Schweitzer as saying, "Anyone who experiences the woes of this world within his heart can never again feel the surface happiness that human nature desires." One can never forget, wrote Schweitzer, the anguished faces of the poor and the sick. Mother Teresa expressed the same view when she said, "Real love is always painful and hurts: then it is real and pure" (p. 105). Such an understanding resonates with the great religious traditions of the world, but it does not sit well with the feel-good morality of contemporary Americans.

Wuthnow draws significant conclusions from the fact that the language of sacrifice has tended to drop out of our vocabulary: "To say that [caring] does not require time and energy, to deny that one can become worn out in doing good, to obscure the fact that real dangers and risks may be necessitated, is simply to lure people into a false understanding of caring that is unlikely to prove enduring. Furthermore, if caring does not entail sacrifice, it may result only in token support that does less for the recipient than it does for the giver" (p. 105).

One rather startling finding of Wuthnow's study is that the single variable that correlates most highly with engaging in voluntary helping activity is knowledge of the parable of the Good Samaritan (Chapter 6, pp. 157–187). He makes no causal argument but just notes the power of narrative in shaping consciousness. Here, too, the news is not all good, for knowledge of this parable declines the younger the cohort. Furthermore, among those over 30, knowledge of the parable is positively correlated with years of education, whereas for those under 30 it is negatively correlated with years of education. While Wuthnow found many who could recount the parable quite accurately, he also found that for others it served as a kind of Rorschach test, revealing more about the consciousness of the subject than the content of the story. As one might imagine, there were more than a few who told of a Samaritan who found a stranger lying injured by the wayside, helped him, and really felt good about himself for doing so. And then there was the version of one informant that tells volumes about our society today: "It is, she says, '[a story] about a gentleman who finds someone by the side of the road and is injured or hurt in some way and he goes to help him and ends up getting injured himself'" (pp. 178–179).

Interestingly, almost all Americans, however accurately they can tell the story, identify with the Good Samaritan. Wuthnow points out that in the early centuries of Christianity it was quite common to identify the self with the traveler beaten and abandoned on the wayside and to see the Good Samaritan as the Christ figure. To see ourselves as caregivers is hard enough; to see ourselves as needing care seems to be even harder.

Having briefly discussed some of the cultural tendencies that endanger practices of caring in our society, I will now address some of the social pressures that have the same negative consequences. The daily press is not always the best source of information about our society, but good journalists often are good sociologists and their observations may on occasion shock us into the recognition of important facts. What follows are the opening paragraphs of a story by Gary Blonston in the *Philadelphia Inquirer* of September 22, 1991:

Whatever white-collar America once assumed about getting ahead, trusting employers or simply staying employed, the reality of the 1990s is becoming clear:
The deal is off.

"There was an implied contract: 'You give us your loyalty, we'll give you security'," says executive-network organizer David Opton of Weston, Conn. "That's not true anymore."

Instead, as corporate America shrinks, consolidates and otherwise cuts costs, it is squeezing more people out of work—and more work out of people—than ever before in the careers of managers, office staff and business professionals.

White collars are proving no more bullet-proof than blue ones. Glass offices are turning out to be fragile fortresses, experience and expertise flimsy weapons. The rules have changed in the office, and as the bulk of the working population moves toward mid-life and midcareer, that means millions of people are feeling uncertainty at a time they had envisioned to be the most secure.

"The recession we're in right now is more than just an economic recession," says Robert Gilbreath, a corporate restructuring consultant in Atlanta. "It's a social and cultural recession."

"There's been a corporate shift in values. It used to be a sign of failure to cut those people. Now it's a sign of corporate machismo. It's gone from a negative to almost a positive."

The German sociologist/philosopher Jurgen Habermas (*The Structural Transformation of the Public Sphere: An Inquiry into a Category of Bourgeois Society*, tr. Thomas Burger, Cambridge: MIT Press, [1962], 1989) has divided institutions into two groups in a way that may help us understand what the *Inquirer* reporter is describing. Habermas speaks on the one hand of the lifeworld (which includes the family, the local community, the church, and the realm of non-governmental public opinion) and on the other hand of the systems (chiefly the market economy and the administrative state). Institutions involved in caring would belong primarily in the lifeworld, but, like other lifeworld institutions, have become increasingly influenced, or, as Habermas puts it when he becomes critical, invaded and colonized by the systems. What Blonston describes as happening in the corporation is today also happening in HMOs and in universities.

Looked at historically, the purpose of the systems is to support the lifeworld, to carry out for the lifeworld more efficiently some of the things that will make the lifeworld better and more fulfilling. The economy and the state are there to serve us, or at least that is what we thought should be the case in a modern democratic society. But problems arise when means become ends, when the instrumentalities that should serve us, should help us live richer lives, actually press us into their service and make us their agents rather than the other way around.

I want to concentrate on the danger to the lifeworld in America that comes from the market economy, as our example of corporate restructuring indicates. We have long been aware of the danger to the lifeworld coming from the totalitarian state. Czeslaw Milosz has spoken of the state, in such societies as Communist Poland, as eating up the substance of society. I want to suggest that the market economy can also "eat up the substance of society." It can "colonize the lifeworld," as Habermas puts it.

Indeed I will argue that the greatest threat to our lifeworld, to real community and to genuine practices of caring, comes not only from a state whose power becomes too coercive (we can never underestimate that danger), but from market forces that become too coercive, that invade our private and group lives and tempt us to a shallow competitive individualism that undermines all our connections to other people. We know that we need to limit the state. I want to argue that we need to limit market forces as well when they become imperialistic and threaten to dominate our lives. Indeed I would argue that there is such a thing as market totalitarianism that parallels state totalitarianism and is a real threat to us in America today.

Since the mid-1970s Americans have been tempted to think that the market economy will provide the freedom that in many ways seems to be slipping away from us in contemporary society. One powerfully influential version of this view comes from the teachings of Milton Friedman and the school of economics he founded, teachings that claim descent from Adam Smith but have lost the moral consciousness that Smith, who spent most of his life as a professor of moral philosophy in Edinburgh, brought to his subject. In the view of Friedman and his successors human beings are exclusively self-interest maximizers, and the primary measure of self-interest is money. It is this philosophy that has been motivating American business for quite some time.

Yet the reality is that American business has not become more competitive, but less so, not stronger, but weaker. In the relentless pressure to think only of the bottom line in the short term the corporation itself has become cannibalized. Unlike our chief competitors,

Germany and Japan, we think less, not more, about how we can include everyone in the corporate culture. Ideology and self-interest combine to create an economy that requires more and more hours of work from more people just to stay even with the cost of living. The real pressures of the job culture and the anxieties they create make it less and less possible for Americans to attend to and care about all those lifeworld structures that make life worth living.

What the relentless effort of Americans to think of human beings as autonomous interest maximizers who also occasionally want to feel good ignores is a truth that most human societies, including our own not so long ago, were quite aware of: namely that human beings are not autonomous atoms, that human beings exist in and through relationships and institutions or they do not exist at all. It is simply absurd to expect a young person growing up amidst violence and poverty, hopelessness and lovelessness, to "just say 'no'" to crack cocaine, without any role model or any institution to support such a personal decision. It is absurd for a government employed psychotherapist on an Indian reservation to diagnose a youth living in a household riven by violence and alcoholism as a "narcissistic personality" in need of psychotherapy, a real example recounted to me by a Native American. Narcissism is a natural response to not being loved and not being cared for and all the psychotherapy in the world will not make up for the absence of a loving family and a loving community—indeed it may only burden the youth with one more demand to solve his problems all alone. T. Berry Brazelton, the well-known pediatrician, claims that he can tell in his child-development clinic at Boston's Children's Hospital which infants at nine months of age already feel a sense of failure. He also says that with the right kind of nurturing such infants can be turned around, can believe in themselves because others believe in them.

Let me turn then from describing the cultural and social structural forces that create a crisis in caring today to some of the recommendations that the authors of *The Good Society* suggest in the conclusion of our book, which we entitled, "Democracy Means Paying Attention."

The Good Society sees serious problems in both our culture and our society. Indeed we have the temerity to call for radical change both in our central values and in our major institutions. But our analysis is less grandiose than that summary implies. Our argument is that the endowment of every one of our institutions, from the family to the nation state, to the international order, is eroding and that the quality of our life is suffering as a consequence. A value system that insists relentlessly on maximizing individual interest does not replenish that endowment but only depletes it, depletes it for the weak at home and abroad and for all future generations. We do not minimize the danger. We would agree with Vaclav Havel that the advanced world is embarked on a course that can only end in what he calls "megasuicide." But we believe what is needed to reverse the course is not some new theory or new plan or new "paradigm" as is so often said, but much simpler things, things that might appear quite naive, such as paying attention.

From the time we were children we were told by our parents and our grammar school teachers to "Pay attention!" Even though we may have grown inured to this injunction and shrug it off, there are few things in life more important. For attention is how we use our psychic energy, and how we use our psychic energy determines the kind of self we are cultivating, the kind of person we are learning to be. When we are giving our full attention to something, when we are really attending, we are calling on all our resources of intelligence, feeling, and moral sensitivity.

While paying attention, attending, is very natural for human beings, our attention is frequently disturbed. One of the most obvious features of psychotics is that they suffer from "disorders of attention" in which they have no control over the thoughts and sensations that come flooding into their minds and cannot consciously decide to focus their attention on objects of their concern. But all of us suffer, though less drastically, from such disorders of attention. When we are doing something we "have to do," but our minds and our feelings are somewhere else, our attention is alienated. In such situations of disordered or alienated attention our self-consciousness is apt to be high. We may suffer from anxiety or, today's common complaint, "stress." Working hard at something we care about, giving our full attention to someone we love—these do not cause stress. But studying a subject we're not interested in and worrying about the grade, or doing things at work that we find meaningless but that the boss requires and we must do if we don't want to lose our job, or just being overwhelmed by more than we can cope with to the point where we feel fragmented and exhausted—these cause stress, these are examples of alienated attention. We attend but fitfully—inattentively, so to speak—and therefore we are not cultivating our selves or our relationships with others. Rather we may be building up strong desires to seek distraction when we have free time.

Unfortunately, many of the distractions we hope will "deaden the pain"—alcohol, restless channel-flipping TV watching, compulsive promiscuity—do not really help, for such distractions too are forms of alienated attention that leave us mildly, or sometimes severely, depressed. We have not exercised the potentialities of our selves and our relationships, and so we have not reaffirmed our selves in the larger contexts that give our lives meaning. If, after a stressful day, we can turn our attention to something that is mildly demanding but inherently meaningful—such as reading a good book, repairing the car, talking to someone we love, or even cooking the family meal, we are more apt to find that we are "relaxed."

Attention is, interestingly enough, a religious idea in more than one tradition. Zen Buddhism, for example, enjoins a state of mindfulness and open attention to whatever is at hand, but Zen practitioners know this is always threatened by distraction. "Each act must be carried out in mindfulness," observes the contemporary Buddhist teacher Thich Nhat Hanh. "Each act is a rite, a ceremony," he writes. "Raising your cup of tea to your mouth is a rite. Does the word 'rite' seem too solemn? I use the word to jolt you into the realization of the life-and-death matter of awareness" (*The Miracle of Mindfulness*, Boston: Beacon Press, 1987, p. 4). Mindfulness is valued because it is a kind of foretaste of religious enlightenment, which in turn is a full waking up from the darkness of illusion and a full recognition of reality as it is.

This idea, common enough in Eastern religions, has analogies in biblical religion as well. God revealed himself to Moses from out of the burning bush as "I am that I am" (Exodus 3:14), and Moses had a hard time getting the children of Israel, distracted by their golden calf, to see the radical truth that had been revealed to him at Sinai. Jesus preached a new reality, a Kingdom of God that he declared was at hand, though most of his hearers could not make it out. Jesus said, "having eyes do you not see, and having ears do you not hear?" (Mark 8:18), but many were too distracted to see or hear. As in the religious examples, we mean to use attention normatively, the sense of "mindfulness," as the Buddhists put it, or "openness to the leadings of God," as the Quakers say.

So far we have considered the issues of attention, of disordered or alienated attention, and of distraction, from the point of view of the individual. Self-control and self-discipline have a lot to do with whether we can engage with life or simply attempt to escape it. But people do not deal with these questions all by themselves, nor can one alone develop a self able to sustain attention. We live in and through institutions. The nature of the institutions we both inhabit and transform have much to do with our capacity to sustain attention. We could even say that institutions are socially organized forms of paying attention or attending, although they can also, unfortunately, be socially organized forms of distraction.

Americans place a high valuation on family life. But if the family is only "a haven in a heartless world," a place that provides distraction from the harshness of the rest of our lives, we are certain to be disappointed. For families require a great deal of attention to function successfully. Despite romantic fantasies, marital love is not a narcotic that soothes all wounds. Attending to each other, expressing our deepest concerns and aspirations and listening to those of the other, are fundamental in a good marriage and crucial to the satisfaction it provides. But if we only expect to be attended to and we don't attend to the other, because we've had too hard a day or whatever, we sow the seeds of marital discord and deprive ourselves of the real rewards of marriage. The fact that married people live longer than single people suggests that marriage provides a kind of attention that is very important for human beings.

Attention is important between marriage partners, but it is fundamental for children. Infants who do not get attention, in the sense of psychic interaction and love, simply cannot survive, even if they are fed and clothed. And the quality of attention that children get has a great deal to do with how they turn out. We have already noted T. Berry Brazelton's work on newborn children to show how important such attention, such care is. In short, I think that attentive homes breed attentive children.

Today there is a crisis with respect to giving and receiving attention in the family. The care of everything and everyone, especially children, is suffering because there is not enough time. Although the solution to this problem involves changes in the larger society, in the short-term there is the immediate obligation on the part of everyone in the family to restore the centrality of attention and care.

But the task of restoring family life, whatever form the family may take, cannot be the family's alone. As Arlie Hochschild has recently pointed out, a "job culture" has expanded at the expense of a "family culture" (*Second Shift: Working Parents and the Revolution at Home*, NY: Viking, 1989). Only a major shift in the organization of work and in American public policy with respect to it will enable us to regain a balance between job and family. It might appear at the moment, when economic competitiveness is such an obsession, that Americans "can't afford" to think about the family if it will in any way hinder our economic efficiency. Nothing could be more shortsighted. In the long run our economic life, like every other aspect of our common existence, depends on the quality of people. How effective will our economy be if it depends on a generation of listless, anxious people unable to concentrate on anything very long and unconcerned with planning a coherent life for themselves? There is literally nothing more important than the quality of our young people, yet American public policy consistently refuses to *pay attention* to this fact.

The current difficulties of the American family have a great deal to do with how isolated it is, geographically and socially. There is much talk about the various "experimental" forms of the family today—two-earner households, single-parent households, same-sex couples with children—as well as "traditional" families where husbands work and wives stay home, but there is a great deal that all these families have in common and that makes it difficult for all of them to sustain family life. As the theologian John Snow ("Families in the Fast Lane to Nowhere," *Episcopal Life*, May, 1990, p. 18) puts it:

> In all these cases the absence of generational rootedness in a certain place with a long term commitment to its community and economic life makes money—cash flow—the primary source of security.
>
> With professional people there is the added security of insurance, health insurance and pensions. For the rest there are welfare, social security and medicare. In all cases the bottom line of security is money, not extended family and community.
>
> For some families there is no bottom line at all. They may be found in shelters, and some of them are healthy young people with small children and no addiction to drugs or alcohol, sometimes with jobs, yet unable to afford rent in such cities as Boston or New York. They lack even an address.

What Snow is suggesting is that stable and attentive families need commitment to a place, which in turn requires locally and regionally coherent economies.

A new look at localism, at decentralization, at what the American philosopher Josiah Royce long ago called "provincialism," in a positive sense, at what Lewis Mumford called "settlement," would be valuable for much more than family life. Localism does not imply any abdication of the responsibility of the federal and state governments for the general population—it does not insist on the devolution of major responsibilities to underfunded and wavering "points of light." But it does envision that the government would support and expand local efforts where they exist—a summer program for teenagers sponsored by a black church in a depressed neighborhood; an effort by workers to buy out and renovate a plant whose owners wished to relocate in Brazil—and also help create such efforts where they don't exist. In Catholic social teaching this is known as the principle of subsidiarity, about which there is some diversity of interpretation. As we use it, subsidiarity implies that higher-level associations such as the state should never replace what lower-level associations can do effectively, but it also implies their obligation to help when the lower-level associations lack resources to do the job alone.

When we think about how money has become so central a measure for everything in our society, including personal worth, and remember that money in most of these contexts is a source of distraction rather than attention, we come face to face with the central paradox of American history. The individual was, in the eighteenth century, embedded in a complex moral ecology that included family and church on the one hand and on the other a vigorous public sphere in which economic initiative, it was hoped, grew together with public spirit. Without overlooking its many injustices, we may note that it was still a society that operated on a humanly intelligible scale. Both the economy and the government were sufficiently small-scale as to be understandable to the ordinary citizen. Looking back from our present position we can see that citizens then were faced with two possibilities, which we may denote as "cultivation" and "exploitation." The pattern of "cultivation" (which we could also call "taking care of") that some Americans for a time did embrace (and others never entirely abandoned) involved the creation of regional cultures in some degree of harmony with the natural environment, where individuals, families, and local communities could grow in moral and cultural complexity. But the temptations of exploitation in so new and so rich a country proved irresistible. Unfortunately, much of the history of the United States is the history of exploitation, not cultivation, exploitation of the American people, exploitation of the North American continent, and exploitation of the world.

The pattern of exploitation was destructive to both the natural environment and the life of the community. It appealed to that aspect of the tradition in which individual accumulation, measured in money terms, came loose from other social goods and became an all-consuming concern, undercutting even the devotion to self-cultivation and the family. And this pattern of exploitation led to the development of large economic and governmental structures that grew "over the heads" of the citizens and beyond their control, making a mockery of the most fundamental principle of American political philosophy: government by the consent of the governed.

We took up the idea of attention as initially a matter of individual psychology. As we followed it, we moved to ever larger social and cultural circles: from self-cultivation, to concern for the family, to our local communities, to our national life and life in the world. Attention and distraction, the disturbance and destruction of attention, occurred at every point. Everywhere attention had to do not only with conscious awareness but with the cultivation of human possibilities and purposes, whereas distraction was a response to fear and exhaustion, leading to shallow escapism in some circumstances, to defensive efforts to dominate and control through power or money in others.

Institutional change comes only as a result of the political process. An attentive democratic politics is not some extraneous demand that busy and harried citizens may ignore or attend to fitfully out of "liberal guilt." Our argument is that if we are going to be the kind of persons we want to be and live the kind of lives we want to live, then attention and not distraction is essential. Concerns that are mostly deeply personal are closely connected with concerns that are global in scope. We cannot be the caring people whom our children need us to be and ignore the world they will have to live in. We cannot hide from the fact that without effective democratic intervention and institution-building the world economy is accelerating in ways that are tearing our lives apart and destroying the environment. Moral discourse is essential in the family; it is also essential in the world. There is no place to hide. It is time to pay attention.

A term closely related to attention in our moral vocabulary is responsibility. Toward the end of the conclusion of *The Good Society* we call on the theologian H. Richard Niebuhr, partly because he absorbed and creatively reworked some of the best social science of his day, to help us think about the social meaning of responsibility. For Niebuhr responsibility is ultimately responsibility to God, although it involves us in a radical relation to the whole world. As he put it:

> In the critical moments we do ask about the ultimate causes . . . and are led to see that our life in response to action upon us, our life in anticipation of response to our reactions, takes place within a society whose boundaries cannot be drawn in space, or time, or extent of interaction, short of a whole in which we live and move and have our being.
>
> The responsible self is driven as it were by the movement of the social process to respond and be accountable in nothing less than a universal community. (*The Responsible Self: An Essay in Christian Moral Philosophy*, New York, Evanston, and London: Harper and Row, 1963, p. 88)

There is a remarkable resonance between the thinking of H. Richard Niebuhr and Vaclav Havel. We feel very close to Havel in some of the things he has been saying. For example, in February of 1990, after he had been President of the Czechoslovak Republic for only three months, in a speech to a joint session of the United States Congress, he said:

> [T]he salvation of this human world lies nowhere else than in the human heart, in the human power to reflect, in human meekness and in human responsibility. . . .
>
> We are still a long way from that "family of man"; in fact we seem to be receding from the ideal rather than drawing closer to it. Interests of all kinds: personal, selfish, state, national, group, and if you like, company interests still considerably outweigh genuinely global interests. We are still under the destructive and vain belief that man is the pinnacle of creation, and not just a part of it, and that therefore everything is permitted. There are still many who say they are concerned not for themselves but for the cause, while they are demonstrably out for themselves and not for the cause at all. We are still destroying the planet that was entrusted to us, and its environment. We still close our eyes to the growing social, ethnic and cultural conflicts in the world. From time to time we say that the anonymous mega-machinery we have created for ourselves no longer serves us,

but rather has enslaved us, yet we still fail to do anything about it.

In other words, we still don't know how to put morality ahead of politics, science, and economics. We are still incapable of understanding that the only genuine backbone of all our actions—if they are to be moral—is responsibility. Responsibility to something higher than my family, my country, my firm, my success. Responsibility to the order of Being, where all our actions are indelibly recorded and where, and only where, they will be properly judged. (*Congressional Record – Senate*, *136*[13], p. S1313)

In the idea of responsibility as Niebuhr and Havel express it, an idea central to a valid notion of care, there is an implicit contrast to what we might call the paradigm of control. If we have learned anything in the twentieth century we have learned that we cannot control the world—not with grand political theories, not with vast wealth, not with overwhelming military power. History is full of surprises. It is just those most devoted to control who are the most dumbfounded—I think of Robert McNamara during the Vietnam War, an almost tragic figure when he had to recognize that his control strategies were leading only to catastrophe. Yet we are ceaselessly called to responsibility, to respond with all our intelligence and wisdom to the new conditions that challenge us. Responsibility does not mean action for its own sake. In one of his letters to his wife Havel points out the foolishness of thinking that when "nothing is happening," nothing is happening. Here I think of Eugene Peterson's admonitions (in this book) about seeming "not to care" because we are recognizing that more is involved than we can control and that sometimes silence and waiting are more important than frenetic action.

I want to end on a note that is shared with my four co-authors, with whom I have worked on two books for the last twelve years, and that note is hope—hope, not optimism. Optimism is based on projections from the big numbers. When I look at the big numbers I am not very optimistic. Hope is related to faith and to responsibility rather than control. Our hope is, of course, shared with millions of others all over the world, and that cannot but be heartening, but it ultimately is based on trust that, against all the odds when we view the world in cold calculating terms, God is good, God is love, Being itself is trustworthy.

NARRATIVE:

Listening to the Heart

LYNN SCHIMMEL

I am a women's health nurse practitioner. My client, Sarah, had already had several years of a difficult marriage when I first met her for an annual exam in the early '80s. She and her husband had much disagreement over whether to ever attempt a pregnancy, but finally did so; a son was born by cesarean due to fetal distress in 1983. Subsequent visits over the next few years found her still feeling unhappy about her life, both with her husband's progressive alcoholism and her own yearning for another baby, which her husband was adamantly against. Sarah's yearning continued to be strong, however, and she became pregnant a couple of years later while using a diaphragm.

The major theme of my interaction with her over the years had been the urging of this fairly nonassertive person to perhaps be more open to her own feelings and respectful of their validity. I don't think it was accidental that she avoided me in the initial appointments regarding this unplanned pregnancy (seeing people in the office who were less familiar with her), until the appointment was already scheduled for a therapeutic abortion. I remember trying to be patient, knowing that she would come to talk with me if and when she wished. She did—the day before the abortion. Our conversation went something like this:

> **Sarah:** I just have to have the abortion. Rick is so angry that I'm pregnant. Our friends don't think it's a good idea either— I'd decided to go through with the pregnancy because I wanted it so much, then Peggy called me at work to tell me that her husband was really mad at me too for making Rick so unhappy. Why can't everybody just leave me alone?
>
> **Lynn:** So I know what Rick wants, and Peggy, and her husband. What do *you* want?

Sarah: I don't know; it's all so confusing. I always wanted a second child, and these children would be a nice number of years apart. But maybe it's not the right thing to do—he's so angry.

Lynn: And you are hurting a lot.

Sarah: I just want the decision to be over! I can't stand feeling like this!

Lynn: I'm sure that this time feels so pressured and awful that *any* decision would seem like a relief, but let me suggest something to you. It has been my experience, watching many people at this stage for varying reasons, that *trying* to make a decision is really counterproductive. What your decision is will become clear to you if you don't try to hurry it, but rather just be with yourself for a little while; you're only 7 weeks pregnant—you have a whole month at least to become peaceful about your decision.

It seems that most people never do get 100 percent for or against having an abortion—the best seems to be about 70/30. If, though, you just *let yourself be* wherever you are at any particular minute or day over the next couple of weeks, I think the roller coaster feeling that women describe will slow down, and it will become clear where your heart mostly is.

During the times you are sure you want to terminate the pregnancy, feel what that would be like—relief, resolution, whatever. On the days you are feeling that you want to continue the pregnancy, let yourself think about everything that surfaces for you then—without any "buts." Just experience as completely as you can what each option would entail. Both sides are real, and both need to have their voice.

After a while, it will become clear where you spend most of your time and your decision can be peaceful, knowing you really examined every possibility on all sides. Letting yourself do that helps us care for the side that didn't "win" later, too—the decision to terminate or continue the pregnancy will care for the 70 percent; but the sadness of the other 30 percent needs care also; spending time with that part now lets us know exactly what you need to grieve for when you say goodbye to that choice.

Sarah said, "I'll think about it." (She wrote later, "I used to talk to the baby and tell it not to worry, that I would not let anything happen to it. I felt so elated when I left Lynn's office—I would be able to do what I really wanted.") Sarah, however, had the abortion the next day, and suffered suicidal ideation in subsequent weeks.

She and her husband planned and achieved a pregnancy the next year; he said that he hadn't comprehended the importance of it to her until after the abortion. That fall, he also was involved in a serious car accident while under the influence of alcohol, and subsequently joined AA. The pregnancy and life progressed uneventfully until 38 weeks when a breech presentation was suspected and so an ultrasound done. The U/S revealed a severe defect, incompatible with life.

I saw her daily the next few days. There were so many issues to deal with—her shock and grief, the guilt she felt for having aborted her last pregnancy, the issue of how to deal with all this with her five-year-old, the preparation of herself and her husband for a probable stillbirth. She cried for hours a day, and I gave her books that kept her crying. We had lengthy discussions about the pros and cons of seeing and holding the baby—I felt so strongly that they should, but, from birthing my own abnormal baby the year before, understood too well their feelings of horror that something so different than what they expected had been growing inside her.

I said to her:

Sarah, I'm so sorry that this is so hard, but there are some things we need to talk about. When Emily is born, those hours will be the only time you will ever have with her. It's important for us to talk about how you want those to be . . . what will you be glad you did many years from now? For example, I remember a woman last year who just wanted to spend one night sleeping curled up with her stillborn baby. These things are done. And though I know you can't even believe we are needing to have a conversation about this, we must.

Sarah answered, "I can't, I can't. I just want this baby. Poor little girl. Why her? Why me?"

The conversation continued haltingly for days. I urged them to take, or allow the taking of, pictures. We decided that at least they might help facilitate their son's grief, which was already surprisingly (to them, anyway) profound. She obsessed about how "bad" the baby might look, and since it was such a rare defect, I had no pictures to help prepare her. I shared with her my feeling that no defect seems as bad when finally confronted as in imagination. I always referred to the baby by her name in our discussions (she had had an amniocentesis and knew the sex), and after initial reluctance, they reverted to this also. Several days later, it was time to go to the hospital. It became clear after a point that labor was not progressing, so another cesarean was done. Emily was, indeed, stillborn. Sarah and Rick held her for hours, dressed her, took many pictures of her, and cried.

I encouraged Sarah to make a baby book that included, among other things, the pictures and a lock of Emily's hair. We also talked frequently in the next few weeks—initially, there were important, obsessive ruminations about exactly when Emily had died and if it was secondary to the procedure that the doctor needed to perform to do the birth, so we got the hospital progress notes and reconstructed this and all the other tiny details that she needed to know to grasp it all. Her five-year-old's reactions were also discussed, and we loaned the family many books from our office library that were helpful for giving words to his anguish as well as their own.

Sarah would say, "I feel like I'm moving away from her so fast. I don't want the days to go by because it moves me farther away from her." And I answered, "Then let's speak of Emily often to help her stay real."

My most important task the next few months was to help her stay in touch with her feelings of sadness that she so wanted to bury. When we talked, I would suggest that she reread some of the books on other parents' experiences of stillbirth as a reminder of how long the process of grieving really takes. When she would make noises about going back to work (which wasn't really necessary monetarily), I'd ask her if she had gone through Emily's things recently and how it had gone, reminding her that that little girl *deserved* a lot of grief. Although I felt almost mean at times about things I would do to help her to stay submerged in the pain that I knew was there, she told me later that staying home the year after Emily's death was the best thing she could have done, as she was "crazy" (her word) with heartache.

It also was important to get the grief worked through as expediently as one can do such things, because she was pregnant again by the end of the year, and so had another little one to work on welcoming.

Helping her stay in touch with both her excitement and terror, especially as the anniversary of Emily's death approached, was the challenge of that pregnancy.

Sarah would say, "Her legs don't move much. Is there a heartbeat? She just doesn't move very much!" I answered, "I think she's fine, but I know nothing is really going to make you feel okay until you're holding a very pink, warm baby in your arms. Why don't you come in every day you want to and listen to her heartbeat—I think it would help a little."

My own bias was for her to attempt a plain old vaginal delivery which, if successful (as 80-90 percent of our VBACs are), would have been powerful for her sense of normalcy and completion. She decided though, at 36 weeks, that she very much preferred a cesarean, saying that she didn't want any more unknowns. I certainly could understand that.

She said, "I feel like I've had two awful experiences—I want to have control over this birth. I know what a cesarean's like; I don't want anything else to think about."

I was there for the birth at her request. Before she became pregnant with this baby, we talked often of the courage and bravery it would take to face living through another pregnancy. I said I could certainly see someone deciding that the pain wasn't worth risking no matter how much another child was wanted. As her perfect daughter was born, that courage was rewarded. I took a million pictures, and we toasted with sparkling apple juice. I was embarrassed at first that they named this little girl after me; "I was only doing my job," as they say. But the naming seemed very important to them, and soon I loved it too.

I overheard her husband telling someone a few weeks later, "Yes, all of our babies were born with a lot of dark hair." The ease with which he said this spoke volumes to me of the work we did incorporating Emily's death into their ongoing life. Also, pictures of Emily's dear face grace their home among other family pictures. Sarah, much later, met a woman who had also had a stillbirth but who, she said, did not have any help processing the enormity of it. She shared the books with her, helped her cry for nearly the first time, and strongly reassured her that, no, she wasn't crazy to be feeling as she did this first year—that her baby deserved a lot of grief. Hearing that Sarah passed on what she had learned from her own anguish was such a tribute to the reality of the ripples of connection that I know extend from every interaction.

The shadows cast, for better or worse, are long. I felt happy we'd created some good ones.

Sarah is struggling now with wanting to work only half-time instead of full-time, but I think she'll be listening to her heart on this. Her husband continues to attend AA successfully, and though they don't have an ideal marriage, they've survived a lot intact. Their son is now six, still occasionally asks to read the "Emily books," and speaks of her in conversation. And I've learned more certainly that it isn't unkind to help someone stay with their grief and listen to their heart.

Caring as a Way of Knowing and Not Knowing

PATRICIA BENNER

An inadequately tapped potential source of spiritual and cultural renewal within an individualistic culture is that individualists have strong moral mandates to respect the rights and dignity of others providing not only freedom from constraints (negative freedom) but also the freedom to realize possibilities (positive freedom). Along with the moral vision of creating individuals who have the "freedom to be all that they can be" we have more subtle, but pervasive skilled caring practices that provide care and teach us how to care in ways that create the strong interdependent "individual" selves. Charles Taylor (1989) identifies three major axes of moral thinking influential in Western societies:

1. the sense of respect for and obligations to others;
2. understandings about what constitutes living a good life;
3. what constitutes human dignity.

"By [dignity] I mean the characteristics by which we think of ourselves as commanding (or failing to command) the respect of those around us" (Taylor, 1989, p. 15). Taylor goes on to note that in our moral heritage we have the specific mandates for recognizing the worth and integrity of all individuals, for universal benevolence and for avoidance of suffering. However, many of our visions of the good life are incongruous and imperiled by the economic and public structures of care. We have systematic patterns of domination and subordination built into our structures of caregiving (Tronto, 1993).

Our public and ethical discourses are constrained by utilitarian individualism, expressive individualism, and ethical discourses based on rights and procedures for ensuring justice (Bellah et al., 1984, and in this volume, pp. 21–27). Our public deliberations on morality are notably silent on the everyday ethical comportment and relationships in caring for one another and raising our young. We have privatized the skills and knowledge embedded in caregiving despite the fact that we have many public institutions for caregiving. As noted in the Preface the large question posed in this work is whether examining our most exemplary caring relationships might prompt us to redesign the structures and processes of our public caregiving institutions to better facilitate caring practices. What can we learn from listening to narratives from the best of our caring practices that will allow us to reconsider the everyday ethical comportment and engaged moral reasoning in these invisible and devalued practices (Dreyfus, 1991)?

This paper examines the moral sources and notions of the good embedded in the public caring practice of nursing, not to claim that nursing in particular is morally superior to any other caring practice. Indeed each caring practice examined in this volume also presents a similar case for the moral sources of socially embedded caring practices. Rather the goal is to point to a more general argument for considering specific caring practices, and narratives from these practices, as visions of liberating, respectful forms of care and as ways of articulating the goods embedded in these practices so that we can more faithfully include caregiving in our public and economic structures. Because I am a nurse, and have studied the caring practices embedded in nursing extensively, I have chosen nursing as an example (Benner, 1984; Benner & Wrubel, 1989). Behind this quest to demonstrate what might otherwise be considered obvious lies the assumption that caring practices continue to be rather invisible, devalued, and typically inadequately accounted for in our institutional designs and public policy.

A practice is a socially embedded organized activity with notions of good inherent in the practice and character of the practitioner (MacIntyre, 1981). Caring practices, dependent on care as a basic mode of being, are constitutive of world and persons in that caring practices allow things and people to be seen and heard. Caring practices (world and person constituting practices) cannot be listed exhaustively but include recognition practices, care of the embodied self, care of children, friendship, participation in a community of concern, care of the frail and ill, teaching, coaching, bearing witness to growth, personhood, triumph and suffering and more (Benner, Wrubel & Phillips, in progress). Parenting, ministering, doctoring, nursing, teaching, psychotherapy, and social work are all socially organized caring practices that allow social space, participation, membership, and dialogue to occur and make being human possible.

Without care, the person is without projects and concerns, is without story. Care sets up a world, and creates meaningful distinctions. Living in a meaningful world is the ground for perceptions and provides concerns and direction for persons. This phenomenological stance departs from theories of motivation based on need satisfaction, or drives, asserting that motivation is based upon concern and caring about specific people, projects, things, and events. Meaninglessness (a place of not caring) and *anomie* (the loss of a feeling of belonging) are the most impoverished coping stances, because nothing stands out as more or less important or inviting for the person (Rubin, 1984; Dreyfus and Rubin, 1991). Nothing really matters. This is the modern vision of freedom from care and attachments. This negative freedom however makes all action look equally plausible and provides no direction for choosing one action over another (Benner and Wrubel, 1989).

Given an atomistic and mechanistic view of the person, care and caring can come to look as if "caring" is a problem or *the* problem. The interdependent caring person cannot claim complete autonomy nor be the absolute center of all meaning giving. This vision of the person runs counter to the dominant quest in the culture for extreme individualism, the quest to be the master of one's own destiny, control all options, including feelings and responses to events. This Cartesian version of untrammeled or negative freedom where the person finally loses all bonds and is free from every care however cannot create the positive freedom to choose and to act even if people were ever really able to be so disconnected (Benner and Wrubel, 1989).

Caring, as defined from a phenomenological perspective, is the most basic mode of being and is central to all helping professions. Caring means that people, interpersonal concerns, and things matter. Caring shapes language and makes questions and issues visible for public debate. Thus, caring sets up the possibility for and is integral to knowing. In health care, caring sets up the possibility for cure. Furthermore, the science and practice of health care workers lose their ethical and epistemologic moorings without an ethic of care and responsibility as a guide (Curtin, 1982; Benner and Wrubel, 1989; Pellegrino and Thomasma, 1988). A strict ethic of rights and justice, with the overriding principle being autonomy, cannot be the primary ethic for nurses or for any health care professional. These claims will be explicated by examining the notions of good embedded in nurses' narrative accounts of expert caring practices.

North Americans confuse care with control. Here I want to suggest that T. S. Eliot's phrase "teach us to care and not to care" (see E. Peterson, p. 68, in this volume) could be translated to "teach us to care and not to control" because doing nothing, sitting on one's hands, resisting the temptation to intervene or take over can be a powerful form of caring for the integrity, dignity, and capacities of the other. When the physician is tempted to rush in, take over, and do intrusive pain-causing surgical interventions, because they are faster, more efficient, and belong to the ethos of mastery, dominance, and control, attentively waiting with caution can be a profound act of care. Effective caregiving requires more than intent or sentiment. It requires skill and knowledge and being in relation with others in ways that foster mutuality, empowerment, and growth.

As those who are wounded and would be helped, and those who would help, I think we are much like the man at the pool of Bethesda, when Jesus came and asked: "Will you be healed?" And the man explained: "You do not understand, I have been sitting by these healing waters for over forty years, and I can get no one to lift me into the healing waters when they are troubled. You will hear sad, and tragic stories today, but I can assure you that mine is the saddest." And if Jesus would have talked to the helping professionals on the scene that day, he might have heard cost benefit calculations and instructions: "Jesus, don't waste your healing time and efforts on that man, it is not cost effective. We have identified his risk factors, he does not have the appropriate motivational profile. You only have so much of the precious bodily juices of healing, therefore you should work with those that we have identified as high potential, this will maximize your success rate, improve your bottom line. We have just introduced a new product line of helpees, attention deficits, and they respond well to help. We have developed a system of identifying high risk and high potential, you'd be smart to only work with that group. You can't help everyone you know. You have to protect your boundaries, you must watch who is touching the hem of your garments."

We, like my imagined modern dialogue with Jesus, have created an industry of excuses for why some people cannot be helped, and why we cannot and must not help them. But fortunately Jesus did not have the benefit of our best professional training. Jesus said to the man: "Take up your bed and walk." And a major portion of this man's healing must have been for him to give up his identity as a victim in order to experience blessing and possibility.

Caring practices are very risky, often paradoxical, always involve connection, mutual recognition, involvement with particular people in particular situations. Because care depends on the receptivity and trust of the one cared for and requires understanding and not just explanation, the knowledge and skill embedded in caring practices are easily overlooked. The language of caring does not easily translate into our public legal and accounting systems since these systems are designed to accommodate business transactions between strangers. In the current "managed competition" and market controls for health care, the focus continues to be on techno-cure rather than the care required to prevent disease and the attentive care that is required to support the consequences of the techno-cure. The cost savings are focused on managing the curative interventions and limiting direct physical and emotional care. This technological way of revealing things has been called "enframing" by Heidegger:

> Only to the extent that man for his part is already challenged to exploit the energies of nature can this revealing that orders happen. If man is challenged, ordered, to do this, then does not man himself belong even more originally than nature within the standing reserve? The current talk about human resources, about the supply of patients for a clinic, gives evidence of this . . . (p. 323). . . . The mode of enframing [ordering for its own sake] is the supreme danger. This danger attests itself to us in two ways. As soon as what is unconcealed no longer concerns man even as object, but exclusively as standing-reserve, and man in the midst of objectlessness is nothing but the orderer of the standing-reserve, then he comes to the very brink of a precipitous fall; that is, he comes to the point where he himself will have to be taken as standing-reserve ([1954] 1993, p. 332).

Drawing on the language of efficiency and standardization, in large-scale organizations, knowledge and skill that cannot be predicted or controlled are discounted. Institutions are caught up with rationalization procedures that can be easily measured in terms of outcomes, economic exchanges and accounting procedures. We have pervasive practices of separating means from ends. We have developed micro-management strategies that rationalize practice through cost controls and statistics about the general case. Our public caring practices related to health care are now lodged in such bureaucracies, managed by even larger insurance bureaucracies. These cost-control strategies have developed in response to runaway health care costs and the recognition that profit motivation is a driving force for cost escalation in a fee-for-service health care system. However, the micromanagement strategies by third-party profit-driven insurance companies cannot legislate skillful ethical comportment on the part of practitioners. Rather they tend to mitigate against engaged ethical and clinical reasoning between practitioner and client. That health care has become a commodity managed by distant payers whose cost control strategies are governed by abstract formulae aimed at maximizing profits is evident in Mahar's (1994) recent economic forecasts for hospitals.

> "Lower margins are inevitable in the hospital industry," [Ed Gordon] acknowledges, "which is why the shrewdest operators are getting out of the hospital business per se and into the business of comprehensive health care." Gordon has completely revised the way he values hospitals. "A hospital operator who thinks of his institution as an acute-care center, delivering medical care and performing surgeries, is headed for Jurassic Park," he declares. "The hospital is instead, becoming a base for technology that may be delivered in someone's home, at a rehab center, or at an alternative site.
>
> "Since hospitals are becoming cost centers, not profit centers, if I were a hospital operator, I'd want an empty hospital. I'd provide as much care as I could more efficiently, in cheaper settings." (Mahar, 1994, p. 17)

This financial account does not consider the cost to the unpaid caregivers in the community who have to assume the care of the acutely ill, nor does it consider the cost for hospitals to deliver highly technical hospital care for the homeless hospitalized as a result of inadequate basic preventive care or those who have no caregivers in the home to provide the intermediate level of care.

Unwittingly the abstract cost controls serve a disease-oriented commodified health care system rather than a system based upon notions of community health promotion, preventive care, reasonable heroics, and humane care. Once the expert clinical and moral reasoning by practitioners who know the patient/family/community are edited out of the system we lose the patient/family control and practitioner expertise. Practicing defensive medicine to avoid lawsuits, and prescribing within the bounds of insurance coverage impinge on patient/family/practitioner clinical/ethical decision making. This market approach tends to substitute techno-cures for caring practices and health promotion. An economic or even narrowly defined "medical outcomes" approach cannot consider what is worth doing (worthy ends) or the larger impact of the health care delivery system on the community.

There are profound differences between a practice, business, and technology. The outcomes of excellent caring practices cannot be reliably predicted in advance and are even dimly understood after they occur. But this does not make them any lesser in their intellectual, moral, aesthetic, skillful knowledge. Expert caring is a way of knowing without the mystery and paradox vacuumed out of it. When nurses are asked what made a particular expert caring relationship possible, the answers typically focus on specific capacities and talents of the care recipient and on the outcomes themselves rather than the traits and talents of the caregiver (Tanner, Benner, Chesla, and Gordon, 1993). A neonatal nurse describes her sense of good work:

> It's very gratifying to have a kid that you've taken care of get well. My primary [infant patient] now started out at 800 grams and he was on the ventilator and he's been very sick. Now he's on full feedings and he's 3 1/2 pounds and he's getting ready to go back to his home town, and he's just a great little kid. And it's so neat after putting all that time into it. It's real wonderful that he gets to the point where you can actually pick him up and carry him around and have him be responsive. That's my gratification. I don't need positive feedback from my peers or letters from my head nurse or any of that. I need to have a kid that looks me in the face and sucks his finger and is doing all the right things. To me that means a lot more than hearing from somebody that thought I did a good charge or something. . . . I really find it gratifying when I have a good day with a patient.

Her rewards are direct and internal to the practice (MacIntyre, 1981). Our abstract accounting systems depend on the ethos embedded in the visions and realizations of excellent practice such as this. Theresa Stephany's (see pp. 120–123) understanding of the human and ethical concerns in caring for her patient who was suspended in unwanted technical interventions is also such an example of the power and effectiveness of engaged clinical and ethical reasoning in the situation. In the situation Ms. Stephany grasped the wife's moral mandate not to take her husband's life. The patient's active refusal of further medical interventions fell within his range of choice and did not violate the ethic of the patient's right to refuse treatment. The nature of this particular clinical and ethical understanding that must be embodied by particular health care practitioners cannot be replaced by policies, procedures, and micro-management. Clinical judgment cannot be sound without knowing the patient's/family's situation and moral concerns. And moral perception cannot be astute without knowing and caring about the patient/family (Tanner, Benner, Chesla, Gordon, 1993).

CARING AS PATIENT ADVOCACY

Nurses have a rich tradition of advocating for patients (Gadow, 1989). This is not a narrow legal sense of advocacy but a much richer form of advocacy that seems closer to the Christian tradition of understanding the Holy Spirit as Advocate, that is one who stands alongside, who interprets, understands and conveys God's presence in the current world. One year in my class of entering Master's students, I found six distinct notions of patient advocacy illustrated by different exemplars labeled as "patient advocacy" by students:

1. *Coordinating and managing the diverse services rendered to the patient so that all the services are organized around an agreed-upon intent that ensures that patient-family well-being.* A nurse who had described clarifying and eliminating conflicting therapeutic goals among diverse medical specialties explained: "I had always prided myself on questioning the uncertain, establishing team goals, pulling everything together in an organized fashion for optimal patient care. I felt that this was a strong component of patient advocacy." This definition of advocacy, making sure that the treatment is coordinated and carried out in line with the patient/family concerns and interests is a common practical understanding of patient advocacy in nursing practice.

2. *Standing in for someone, giving them their own voice.* This too is a common form of patient advocacy as understood by nurses. Nurses often hear delicate stories of care and fragility from family members and help them speak these messages to one another. When this fails, they, with permission, will speak the difficult for a family member. "I spoke for the father to the son dying with leukemia. Your father understands that you are dying, he can let you go now. It's O.K., you can relax. You can let go, you can die."

   The father could not say this directly to the son, but through the nurse's advocacy could be with the son and could acknowledge that he could let go. Another nurse describes doing a home visit for a woman after a stroke had confined her to a wheelchair. Finding that the two male caretakers in the household had not understood her feelings, she voiced for the woman: "You must be very angry. It must be awful to have people tell you what to do, and not be able to do these things yourself." This enabled the woman to cry and opened the doors of understanding of the husband and brother caregivers.

3. *Getting the caring needed for significant losses and meanings.* Often caregiving is inappropriate or not attuned because of a lack of understanding of the other's situation. In a very difficult situation where a mother was confronting the death of her infant son, a psychiatrist and assistants had come to take the distraught mother away for acute crisis intervention. Entering the situation, the psychiatrist was unaware of the mother's situation, and the intervention was ill-timed. The mother had not yet spent enough time with the son. The nurse intervened: "I looked up and listened to the psychiatrist as he tried to explain to the mother why she needed to be hospitalized. He requested that she say good-bye to the baby and come with them. He offered to place the baby back in the crib. She was immediately resistant. 'Please' I interjected: 'She has just lost her son.' This advocacy was enough to allow the mother the time she needed with her son. Here by advocacy, the nurse means understanding the other's situation, standing alongside the other, and presencing oneself, strengthening the other's ability to be seen and heard.

4. *Getting the appropriate medical intervention for the patient.* Getting the medical help needed is also a common understand-

ing of patient advocacy. This definition was evident in numerous exemplars about providing an early warning signal to other health care team members, getting an appropriate physician response; or providing and ensuring adequate health care. This form of advocacy blends understanding and interpretation and ensures that patient/family rights and interests are served. Often aspects of the medical situation have been overlooked or misinterpreted and, as advocate, the nurse brings the situation up for review and clarification.

5. *Caring for the dying.* Nurses also call presencing and acknowledging loss and grief "patient advocacy." Here they are drawing on advocacy as a form of understanding. Because dying is segregated and denied in this culture, nurses often consider advocating for the concerns, experience, and rights of the dying to die with dignity. The goal is to have death as a human passage acknowledged and to prevent undue suffering from futile intrusive therapies. Understanding and advocating for comfort care for the dying takes moral imagination and skilled know-how.

6. *Holism.* Patient advocacy is also understood as a form of caring for the whole patient, attending to the illness and its human significance. By attending to the projects interrupted by illness experience, concerns, and implications, the nurse considers that she/he is advocating for the care of the person, and not just the disease process. This form of advocacy provides links to the concerns and community of the person in the midst of breakdown and illness.

In our culture responsibility and blame are part of the illness discourse. Informally we hold a Cartesian view that the mind can control the body, through healthy emotions, life-style, self-care, preventative medical care, etc. Self acceptance is hard won when the body is not "controlled" by the mind and one believes in mind over matter. The oppositional relationship of mind with body extends to self with other. Therefore one incurs intolerable debts by asking for and receiving help. This too is a way in which advocacy for the patient includes self-understanding and acceptance (Benner, Janson-Bjerklie, Ferketich, and Becker, 1994).

That patient advocacy is dependent on openness and engaged moral and clinical reasoning is evident in the following exemplar by nurse Kim Baird:

"Sammy"
Kim Baird, R.N.

"Sammy." I'm sure I will carry his face, his name, his story with me for a very long time; maybe forever. Sammy was a 6 year old Amish boy who had the misfortune of being on the bad side of a particularly nasty mule on the family farm. The injury he received when the mule's foot met his cranium left him with a skull fracture the neurosurgeon described as a "jigsaw puzzle of slivers," brain lacerations/contusions and profound cerebral edema.

Sammy had spent days in Pediatric Intensive Care Unit after his craniotomy for the repair of his head injury. He was ventilator-dependent much of that time. He was transferred to the floor at the end of my shift on Friday with a Keofeed tube in place and a horseshoe shaped incision on the right side of his head. Like most head injury patients, he was extremely combative and needed constant restraints to prevent injury to himself or dislodgement of his tube. "Great weekend ahead," I thought grimly, eyeing this latest addition to an already busy group of patients.

Unfortunately for Sammy and his family, the damage done to his brain tissue was extensive. The physician had told his parents the best they could hope for was a child who could take food orally. Sammy would never walk or talk. He would always be completely dependent on them.

Saturday morning began auspiciously enough. As I made walking rounds with the 11 P.M. to 7 A.M. nurse, we found Sammy's mother already dressed, knitting quietly at his bedside. Sammy had somehow wiggled out of his restraints and had pulled out his Keofeed—it lay next to him in bed. "Nice start," I thought to myself—confirming my fear of what the weekend would hold. The Amish, as a group, are a quiet, reserved sect, not given to emotional outbursts. Although I feel I usually handle parents well, particularly in a time of crisis, I found it difficult to spend any extra time in Sammy's room—not because of him, but because of the quiet, accepting, *waiting* manner of his mother. Having a daughter myself, I found it difficult to reconcile her seemingly passive acceptance of their tragedy and what

I was positive would have been certifiable lunacy on my part, had I been in her shoes.

Except for the predictable diarrhea so common in patients with bolus naso-gastric tube feeds of Ensure, Saturday passed without further incident. Sammy's mother did much of his care, changing his diaper, bathing him, helping me turn him without letting his free hand grab his tube. Her touch was always gentle and loving, but her quietness continued to disturb me.

Sunday started out better. Sammy's mother explained that the family would be going to church but that Sammy's older sister would stay with him. The sister, she explained, spoke English and Dutch and would be able to translate if Sammy needed anything. The fact that Sammy hadn't made an intelligible sound in *any* language didn't seem to figure into her thinking at all.

Just after lunch, the call light over Sammy's door went on. The voice of his sister over the intercom confirmed my worst fear—"Sammy pulled his tube out." As I walked to his room, I mentally tallied the people who might be available to help hold Sammy while the resident replaced the Keofeed and during the subsequent X-ray to check tube placement. In his room, it was just as I had anticipated—the tube lay in his bed and his sister was vainly trying to prevent him from shredding his diaper—a lost cause.

I talked to him as I began to untie his remaining restraints and change his diaper. What I said is not important, probably something trivial like "Sammy, what are we going to do with you?" But, as I spoke, I looked at him and felt for the first time since I'd been caring for him, that he was looking at me—not the vacant wild-eyed look I'd grown accustomed to, but an understanding, "with-it" gaze I had not seen before.

I thought about the standing order on his Kardex: "May try P.O. fluids." We had all laughed about that—Sammy had no swallow or gag reflex at all. As I looked at him, remembering the struggles of replacing the tube the previous days, I thought: "Why not? Let's give it a try." I told his sister I was going to try to give Sammy a drink by mouth. She looked somewhat skeptical, but didn't say anything. I cranked his bed up, left his restraints hanging at the sides and filled a Dixie cup with water from the sink. I cannot describe the feeling that came over me as that child *gulped* down that 60 cc. of plain old tap water—the fluttering of my stomach, the pounding of my heart, the shortness of my breath. And, when I went to refill the cup, Sammy spoke.

Even if I could pronounce or understand what he said, I could not reproduce it here because Sammy spoke in Dutch. But, even to my ignorant ear, it was evident that this 6 year old was demanding something. His sister's eyes opened wide as she looked from him to me and said: "He would rather have iced tea." To this day, I think I flew to the kitchen to get Sammy some iced tea. After an additional 150 cc. went down without incident, I decided he was ready to advance. I called his resident to ask if he could have some ice cream. I am reasonably sure the resident thought I'd lost my mind or was chemically impaired— they all knew Sammy had still been a "neurologic nothing" on the morning rounds. But he said I could try—"Just don't let him aspirate, he goes to the rehabilitation center tomorrow."

I returned to Sammy's room and (unthinkingly) asked his sister if vanilla would be all right. I was only two steps up the hall when she came after me. "He says he'd rather have chocolate." It was only a short time afterwards that Sammy's family returned from church. In that time, I was just thrilled at the progress he made—even *walking* to the bathroom with minimal assistance to void in the toilet. I wondered how his mother would react when she returned.

Not only his parents, but grandparents, siblings, aunts, and uncles came to see Sammy that day. The reserve they have never lifted—as Sammy's grandfather said: "This is God's way"—but the excitement in the room was palpable. And, the two tears that glistened on his mother's cheeks when Sammy spoke to her in Dutch told me that inside, Sammy's mother was shouting her joy from every rooftop.

The conclusion to Sammy's story is that several weeks later, after a stay at a nearby rehabilitation center, Sammy came back to see me—walking, talking Dutch with his family, and shy, as many 6 year olds are with people they don't know that well. His mother thanked me for the care Sammy had received and said how wonderful all the doctors and nurses had been. Her praise made me feel more than a little ashamed. After all, we were the ones who had pooh-poohed the oral fluid order. I had mentally cringed at the idea of letting Sammy's sister be at his bedside as an interpreter because we all "knew" he would never speak again. But these people with their quiet faith, despite what must have been a terrible heartache for them, had believed in their God, in Sammy, and in us.

The significance of this event in my professional life is multifaceted. First, it made me examine myself and the way I deal with others—particularly the quiet parent. Even though it may be uncomfortable, I make myself take extra time to talk to that quiet mom or dad. Often that reserve is a facade of their inner terror. Although they appear to be coping, a few gentle, nonthreatening questions about the kids at home, their jobs, or some trivial chitchat can open them up, allowing them to express their fears, thoughts, and questions.

The second area of significance has to do with labels. Although we are taught as nursing students that labels such as "slow" or "retarded" can become self-fulfilling prophecies, I do not think that concept fully impacted on me until that day. So now, even though I do not always succeed, I make the extra effort to orally feed a baby with a gastrostomy tube looming in her future or extra hard to teach a mom who has difficulty grasping the importance of Digoxin and Lasix therapy for her child. Labels, as I found out, can be misleading and can dull good nursing sense.

Finally, this event is most significant because I regard it as something of a miracle. Having worked on pediatrics for six years, I know physicians give the parents an optimistic but realistic prognosis, if possible. To hear their pronouncement for Sammy signified that this was indeed a sad situation. I've since heard other parents talk about their "miracle baby" or the "miracle" that happened to their child and I have to think there is an intangible something in human beings—faith in the God of their choice, the essence of the human spirit, an inner drive's obvious source. This is what keeps me at this difficult, wonderful job— helping these children physically, hoping that their "miracle" will come through for them. On those long days when every I.V. is blown and every resident is in a foul mood, the miracle and triumph of Sammy can still make me smile. (1991, pp. 5–7)

This narrative is a moral discourse, an example of learning ethical comportment within a practice. Generosity and mercy triumph over a deficit normative or procedural account concerned only with meeting minimal standards of conduct for rights and justice or injustice. Iatrogenesis or the possibility of a lawsuit do not loom in the background of this moral discourse, rather it is propelled by how "true" the nurse is to the particular demands of the situation. A dialogue on how to be true to this moral instruction is taken up in Baird's subsequent nursing practice. But the experience provides more than new information: it is transformative, providing a source of moral imagination and a sense of possibility that give integrity and value to her work. Her memory of the experience actively engages her embodied skilled know-how complete with feelings that allow her to recognize similar situations and possibilities in the future. Strategic language takes a back seat to significance language. The "experience" doesn't turn the nurse into a believing Amish, but it does enlarge her moral imagination to include the ways of being that she can now recognize in the Amish community. She translates their "faith" experience into her secular world but leaves room for the somewhat incommensurable world she has encountered. The concrete example of healing and self-transcendence in the Amish community that sustains her in difficult times "makes it all worth while, and can bring a smile to her face." Future clinical situations are interpreted or understood in light of this experience that I would characterize as a constitutive, and sustaining narrative (Benner, 1991).

NARRATIVES OF EXPERIENTIAL LEARNING AS ETHICAL DISCOURSE

This is an example of a narrative of healing and transcendence that this nurse understands as constitutive and sustaining. In other words, the experience described in the narrative gave her a new understanding of the significance of her work, and this vision sustains her connection and confidence in the worth of her work. Other examples of plots or themes that are illustrative of constitutive and sustaining narratives are:

1. The heroic saving of a life through skillful quick action and the appropriate use of technology, or as characterized by nurses in a small group interviews as a "real save" where the person returns to a full life. (Lives saved inappropriately so

that prolonged dying occurs are excluded, indeed are the feared opposite.)

2. Fostering care and connection between patient and loved ones, or patient and nurse. Often this occurs with premature infants in neonatal intensive care units, but it also occurs frequently with families of adult patients who are extremely compromised.

3. Stories of presencing or not abandoning patients.

These stories depict the difficulty of fidelity in the midst of suffering. A dramatic example is the communication, touch, and connection with a patient suffering from a "locked in" syndrome where there is conscious awareness but no motor ability to communicate except perhaps by blinking the eyes (Benner, Wrubel and Phillips, In Progress). Exploring the concrete examples of constitutive and sustaining narratives can help us articulate the best of our practice and consider how we might better design our caregiving structures and processes, including our accounting procedures to better facilitate this work.

Stories of Exclusion, Objectification, and Defense

Some situations lie beyond the nurse's understanding. They are abhorrent and unapproachable and produce stories of dismay, exclusion, objectification, and defense in order to deal with the terror of the suffering, pain, or even evil. These stories provide outside-in accounts rather than engaged narratives and they have no common themes of caring practices. It is important to tell and hear these stories because they present a moral agenda for the practitioner and the community.

When caring practices deteriorate, stories of rejection, dominance, control, and power struggles are heard. The stance is one of objectification and disengagement and fits the descriptions of "burnout" or loss of human caring (Maslach, 1982). From this disengaged stance the other shows up as wholly other with no common humanity, and the narrative does not take the form of transformation or learning.

The loss of story

Stories of rejection and anger are more engaged than extreme indifference that creates a loss of narrative memory for particular stories. In a study of clinical nursing expertise (Rubin, 1994) some nurses could not remember any particular patients/families and literally could not tell any stories from their practice. They would respond to requests for stories with responses like: "I cannot tell you what I do in particular, I can tell you what I do in general." When pressed for an account of the current day, they would offer descriptions of what they had done rather than stories of care of particular patients/families. They had become technicians doing tasks rather than practitioners engaged in care and restoration. It is not hard to understand why practice would deteriorate to this "job description" level given the overwork and institutional press for efficiency and the societal taboos against getting "too involved." These nurses were not considered expert nurses by their peers even though they had been working for five or more years. I interpret the loss of narrative memory as an indication of lack of involvement with particular patient/families. This loss of engagement and loss of narrative memory is encouraged by the loss of public space for narrative accounts of patient care and diminished shared dialogue between practitioners.

The Practice of Storytelling

Public storytelling among practitioners allows for noticing distinctions and clinical learning. The forming of the story, where it begins, how it develops, what concerns shape the story and how the story ends as well as the dialogue and perceptions of the storyteller present meaningful accounts of practical engaged reasoning (Rubin, 1994). The narrative reveals what is significant and relevant to say about situations and events in the practice. The storyteller can be surprised by the way the story is formed and unfolds because the lived experience can take over the storyteller's account in its immediacy. To tell one's story is also to hear one's story. Storytelling is more immediate than formal procedural or analytical accounts usually presented in formal documents or case presentations by professionals. The structure of the story, the chronology, asides, and the remembered dialogue can reveal assumptions, and taken for granted meanings of which the storyteller is only dimly aware. In presenting the paths chosen, one can reflect on the paths and options that were not taken, even the ones that did not occur to the person at the time. Thus, storytellers, hearing their own stories, can learn from them. The listener can enrich and augment what is heard and understood by the storytelling. Dialogues can be created between others and one's own stories.

Narratives and narrative knowing allow us to examine practical moral reasoning and to get beyond abstractions. Real stories keep us honest and penetrate our systems of rationalizations. Stories require that we open ourselves to mystery, paradox, courage, and wisdom. We are afraid that compassion will be excessive, ill-guided and expensive; we have overlooked the stories that tell us that compassion can be wise, and while costly in human terms, in the long run be less costly than "defensive" adversarial commodified techno-cure. If we were able to replace our disease care system with caring practices that foster illness prevention and health promotion so that clinical wisdom could be fostered for caregivers and receivers alike, we would alter dramatically how we are spending our health care dollar.

If health care workers challenged their preoccupation with pathology and deficits and focused on wholeness, and on what creates wholeness, our therapies and structures for health care would change. As we more clearly see what we have created we can free ourselves to create new visions for our health care systems.

In sum, we need not just a reform of the health care system but a transformation:

Those that would bring healing and be healed have lost their place
    to stand.
We no longer understand our society, community, family,
    our spirit as sources of healing.
We have a strange and estranged relationship with suffering.
We use it as a tool of pity, a source of blame, or experience
    it as a terrible embarrassment, a failure, a momentary break-
    down of control—the technological promise.
We have colonized sickness, and made it an industry of
    assessment, diagnosis, and deficit accounting;
    we give little attention to our healing arts.
We are like the man at the pool of Bethesda when asked by Jesus
    if he would be healed; we offer excuses and reasons why we
    cannot make it to the healing waters.
We prefer despair over freedom, understanding "freedom" as
    dis-connectedness, disengagement, unencumberance.
Freedom from instead of freedom to be and to be with others.
We have made recovery a never ending project
    instead of an epiphany, a new beginning.

We do not understand how to be taught, healed
    and comforted in our suffering.
Like ourselves, our health too has become a possession to be
    used, but seldom a place of teaching,
    an occasion of courage and healing.
We grasp it making it an altar of self-pity and secondary gains
    We have made "being healthy" a career
    and have forgotten its giftedness.
We have forgotten how to come together as communities of
    concern rather than competing individuals who forget that we
    all are needy at times.
We have covered over our embodied capacities and limitations.
We seek to transcend our bodies rather than respect and live
    within our bodily capacities and limitations.
We have lost our stories of healing.
We have lost our stories of suffering.
We have lost our stories that create us, sustain us and bind us
together as supplicants and celebrants.
We have colonized health, and lost our ability to rejoice in it,
    protect and preserve it.
We need a new vision of health and well being.

                                                      (Benner, 1992b adapted)

REFERENCES

Baird, K. (1991) "Sammy" in Benner, P. (1991) "The role of experience, narrative, and community in skilled ethical comportment." *Advances in Nursing Science.* 14 (2)1–21.

Bellah, R. et. al. (1984) *Habits of the heart.* Berkeley, CA: University of California Press.

Benner, P. (1984) *From novice to expert: Excellence and power in clinical nursing practice.* Menlo Park, CA: Addison-Wesley.

Benner P. and Wrubel, J. (1989) *The primacy of caring, stress and coping in health and illness.* Reading, Mass: Addison-Wesley.

Benner, P. (1991) "The role of narrative, experience and community in ethical expertise." *Jo. Advances in Nursing Science.*

Benner, P., Tanner, C., Chesla, C. (1992, a) "From beginner to expert: Gaining a differentiated world in critical care nursing. *Advances in Nursing Science* 14(3), 13–28.

Benner, P., (1992b) "Lamentations" *Journal of Christian Nursing.* 9 (3) 9–11 adapted.

Benner, P., Janson-Bjerklie, Ferketich, S., Becker, G. (1994) "Moral dimensions of living with a chronic illness: Autonomy, responsibility and the limits of control." in *Interpretive phenomenology: Embodiment, caring and ethics in health and illness.* Benner, P. (ed.) Newbury Park, CA.: Sage Publishers.

Benner, P., Wrubel, J., Phillips, S. (in progress) Critical caring, helping practices of critical care nurses. A book length manuscript (1994).

Curtin, L. (1982) The nurse patient relationship: Foundation, purposes, responsibilities and rights. In *Nursing ethics: Theories and pragmatics.* L. Curtin, M. J. Flaherty (eds.)

Dreyfus, H. L. (1991) *Being in the World: A commentary on Being and Time, Division I.* Cambridge, Mass.: MIT Press.

Dreyfus, H. L., Rubin, J. (1991) Appendix: Kierkegaard, Division II and later Heidegger. In Dreyfus, H. L. (1991). *Being-in-the-world: A commentary on Being and Time, Division I.* Cambridge Mass: M.I.T. Press.

Gadow, S. (1989) Clinical subjectivity: Advocacy with silent patients. *Nursing clinics of North America 24* (2)535–541.

Heidegger, M. (1962) *Being and time.* Macquarrie, J. and Robinson, E. (trans) New York: Harper & Row.

Heidegger, M. (1954, 1993 trans.) The question concerning technology. in *Martin Heidegger, Basic Writings.* D. F. Krell (ed.) First translated by William Lovitt, 1977, revised by D. F. Krell. New York: Harper and Row, pp. 323 & 332.

MacIntyre, A. (1981) *After virtue.* Notre Dame, IN: University of Notre Dame Press.

Mahar, M. (1994) "Tomorrow's hospital for profit or not, it will be radically different. *Barron's National Business and Financial Weekly,* January 1994, p. 17 [pp. 12–18].

Maslach, C. (1982) *Burnout-the costs of caring.* Englewood Cliffs, New Jersey: Prentice-Hall.

Pellegrino, E. D. & Thomasma, D. C. (1988) *For the patient's good.* New York: Oxford University Press.

Rubin, J. (1984) *Too much of nothing: Modern culture and the self in Kierkegaard's thought.* An unpublished dissertation, University of California, Berkeley.

Rubin, J. (In Press) "The role of qualitative distinctions in acquiring clinical and ethical expertise." A contribution in *Expertise in nursing practice: caring, clinical judgment, and ethics* Benner, P, Tanner C., Chesla, C. New York: Springer.

Tanner, C., Benner, P., Chesla, C., Gordon, D. (1993) "The phenomenology of knowing a patient." *Image: Journal of Nursing Scholarship. Vol. 25* (4) 273–280.

Taylor, C. (1985) *Philosophical papers. Vols. I. & II.* Cambridge: Cambridge University Press.

Taylor, C. (1989) *Sources of the self: The making of modern identity.* Cambridge, Mass: Harvard University Press.

Taylor, C. (1991) *The ethics of authenticity.* Cambridge, Mass.: Harvard University Press.

Taylor, C. (1992) "The politics of recognition," in *Multiculturalism and "The politics of recognition."* editor, A. Gutmann. Princeton, NJ: Princeton University Press.

Taylor, C. (1993) Explanation and practical reason. in *The Quality of life.* M. C. Nussbaum and A. Sen (editors). Oxford: Clarendon Press.

Tronto, J. (1993) *Moral boundaries, A political argument for an ethic of care.* New York: Routledge.

NARRATIVE:

Meeting at the Table

DOUGLASS E. FITCH

I became the pastor of Downs Memorial United Methodist Church on July 1st, 1987, after having spent the preceding seventeen years studying, being an administrator in higher education, and serving as an assistant to two bishops in two separate annual conferences of the United Methodist Church. In 1986 I said to my bishop, "I need to be in the local church. My spirit is drying up, and I just need to be where people are who desire preaching, pastoral care, and a teaching ministry."

My prayers were answered. Bishop Leontyne T. C. Kelly, the first African-American female bishop in the history of my church appointed me to serve as the pastor at Downs. As soon as I arrived at the church, I encountered my first pastoral care situation. A telephone call came to the church office during my second or third week at the church. Mrs. Ambrosia Jones was home from the hospital following surgery for cancer. I did not know her condition. All I knew was that she was home.

I looked through the membership roster and found her address. The office had older pictorial directories that gave me a picture, though not a very recent one, of the woman I was to see. Much time, fifteen to seventeen years, had passed since I had made my last home visit; I was anxious. My secretary did her best to prepare me for the visit, but the "ball" was in my court.

With my secretary's excellent directions I found the home of Mrs. Ambrosia Jones. My knock on the door was answered by a woman in her twenties. She escorted me to her grandmother's—Mrs. Jones'—room. Mrs. Jones thanked me profusely for coming and expressed her profound thanks to God for getting her through a difficult surgery. It was then that I learned her cancer was not terminal.

Our conversation was going more smoothly than I had expected when Mrs. Jones abruptly stopped speaking. She looked agitated and then called to her granddaughter to bring her a meal. The grandmother

63

and granddaughter began to argue. Remember that this was my first home visit in seventeen years. I felt awkward and began to think that the arguing was not good for either of the women, especially for the recovering grandmother. As the argument went on, I began to see the granddaughter as callous and insensitive. Clearly, the two of them had a lot of history between them; nevertheless, I thought the argument was inappropriate at this time. I did not interrupt their argument, and eventually the granddaughter left the house without preparing the meal.

When Mrs. Jones and I were alone, I tried to assuage her fears about her granddaughter by assuring her that she would return. I offered to speak with the young woman if Mrs. Jones approved. She accepted my offer, and she cried while telling me about how she and her husband had sent the granddaughter to the best schools, sent her abroad, and cared for her every need. While she struggled to recover from a frightening, exhausting surgery, Mrs. Jones was also heartbroken over her granddaughter.

I asked Mrs. Jones if I could pray with her and read some scripture. She said, "Yes. Please do!" I read the passage from the letter to the Corinthians in which Paul writes about our bodies being "earthen vessels." The passage had words about being hemmed in but not forsaken, knocked down but getting up again and again.

Following the scripture reading and prayer, it was clear to me what I was to do. I asked her, to her surprise and mine, "What do you have in your kitchen that you can eat and would like to eat?" She exclaimed, "Oh, Reverend, no! I'll wait for my son or daughter to come by." I said, "It might be a long time of waiting and in your condition you can't afford to miss any meals. If you are hungry, you need to eat right now. And, besides, I didn't get married until I was twenty-seven years old. This preacher knows how to cook. I cook meals during the week for my own family. It's time for you to order! So order up right now!"

As it turned out, Mrs. Jones could not eat much. I fixed soup, a salad, and a sandwich, which were mostly uneaten. But during our time together she told me a great deal about herself. Her life was fascinating. She was the first African-American woman to own and run a travel agency in northern California and the first African-American woman to own a beauty college west of the Mississippi. She was widowed when her husband died of a heart attack after an employee embezzled $300,000 from them. Her grandfather was Edward Wysinger who, in the early 1800s, petitioned the courts to admit black people to public education. He won the case, and it was the Wysinger Law that effectively enabled black people to enter public schools in California.

Hearing Mrs. Jones tell her family history made me see that she was a woman whose strength had been forged in the crucible of life. Her strength became a reservoir from which I asked her to draw during this time of recovery.

After her recovery, Mrs. Jones attended church services with her granddaughter and grandson. She has not missed more than two worship services in almost five years. She is a strong support to her pastor and her family, and she is a strong believer in the power of prayer. She helped this re-tread pastor get started in a new and fresh way in my ministry at Downs. If I have any strengths at all in preaching, pastoral care, teaching, and outreach, it is because people like Mrs. Ambrosia Jones helped me get my priorities straight when I first arrived at the church.

Teach Us to Care and Not to Care

EUGENE H. PETERSON

Pastors set up shop at the corner where the ways of men and women and God intersect. Most people seem to show up at this crossroads lost or discouraged or fatigued or confused. The task of the pastor assigned to this intersection is to give direction to people on the way, encourage and exhort them, provide information about weather and road conditions, serve up refreshments.

It is an incredibly busy place, traffic hurtling this way and that. There are a lot of accidents and injuries, and therefore much caring to be done. It goes without saying that pastors are involved in matters of care. Baron von Hugel used to say, "Caring is the greatest thing; Christianity taught us to care." Pastors care—and if they don't, they don't stay in business long.

The word is at the heart of our tradition. *Cura animarum*, the cure of souls, combines meanings that have separated into words cure and care: cure—nurturing a person toward health; care—being a compassionate companion to a person in need. Cure requires that we know what we're doing; care requires that we be involved in what we are doing. Applied knowledge is necessary but not enough. Empathetic concern is necessary but not enough. *Cura* contains both dimensions, curing and caring.

But getting the word right doesn't ensure right practice, as is obvious when we look around us. There is a huge irony here; we know more about caring than any generation in the history of humankind, we have more men and women professionally trained in the skills of caring and committed to a professional life of caring, yet the reports coming back day after day from the field—people telling stories of what happened to them in the hospital, in church, with the social worker, at school—document an alarming deterioration in care on all fronts. Instead of being cared for people find themselves

66

abused, exploited, organized, bullied, condescended to, and ripped off. There is nothing new in this, of course. People in the need of care show up in a weakened condition, and such vulnerability always seems to arouse the killer instinct in a few individuals who use their professional roles as cover to indulge themselves in one or several of the deadly sins. For thousands of years now bitter stories have been told of the rapacity of priests and physicians, nurses and counselors as they move smilingly through our communities in their sheep's clothing. Dante and Chaucer between them pretty much covered the rascality dimensions in their stories. There is not much more to be said on those aspects of the crises in care. And there is nothing much more to be done on it except set a few watchdogs and catch them when we can.

The crisis that we are concerned with seems to me to develop out of a quite different condition, not an epidemic of criminal conduct among the caring professionals, but something more subtle and pervasive, and far more likely to involve the well-intentioned rather than the ill-willed. In order to do something about it, it is not enough to get rid of a few bad eggs in our respective professions. Something like a renovation of the imagination is required—a re-visioning of who we are and what we are doing that recovers the largeness and health, the essential sacredness of all vocational caring that develops out of our Christian and Jewish communities of experience.

I would like to take a few steps back and get a running start on this by taking a text from T. S. Eliot's poem *Ash Wednesday.* The text is "Teach us to care, and not to care. Teach us to sit still."

Eliot qualifies as a preacher to be reckoned with in these matters because he both lived through and then articulated in prophetic oracles much of what we are dealing with. In the poem that made him famous, *The Waste Land*, he showed the chaos and aridity of a world without God, without community, without traditions. It was the world that Nietzsche had campaigned for under his slogan "God is dead." But Eliot not only wrote this world into recognition, he lived it. *The Waste Land* was also within him and he went over the waterless, treeless ground day after day. His marriage consigned him to continual humiliation and guilt. His alienation from family and country cut him off from emotional nurture and an organic sense of place. And then he became a Christian. His conversion was a scandal among the cultured despisers, a betrayal of the new religion of sophisticated despair for which he had written the canonical scriptures. He worked his emerging Christian faith and hope into the lines of poetry even more skillfully than he had his unchristian skepticism and despair. After *Ash Wednesday,* he went on to the *Four Quartets,* the greatest poem of faith in our century. In these poems that arise out of the world of the wasteland, Eliot searches out fragments of truth, gathers up shards of tradition that are scattered up and down our streets and alleys by the wrecks and collisions caused by God-ignorant and soul-denying drivers and puts together by prayer and poetry a witness to a world that, because of God's creation and redemption, is a garden, a rose garden in fact, and not a wasteland, no matter how frequently and learnedly journalists and scholars report it as a wasteland.

The primary reason that there is a crisis in caring is because it is being carried out on the mistaken presupposition that caring takes place in a wasteland. If we are going to free ourselves from the mistaken wasteland presupposition we must re-learn the world. Since Eliot explored this wasteland as thoroughly as anyone in our century, and in the process found his way by prayer and penitence into a garden, he seems to me to be a good guide, and his text a focused prayer for our enterprise here: "Teach us to care, and not to care."

TEACH US TO CARE

We begin with a realization of poverty: We don't know how to care. What we have been prayerlessly engaged in and glibly calling care is not care. It is pity, it is sentimentality, it is do-goodism, it is ecclesiastical colonialism, it is religious imperialism. Caring, noble and commendable as it seems, is initiated by a condition that can and often does twist it into something ugly and destructive.

The condition is need. A child cries out, a woman weeps, a man curses, a youth, as we say, "acts out." More often than not, there is someone there to help, to care. Sometimes that person is a pastor. So far so good. The child's pain, the woman's tears, the man's anger, the youth's confusion are all real enough. If someone is there, available and willing to care, it is counted as sheer blessing.

But there is another element in the scenario that is frequently missed, and when missed silently and invisibly squeezes all the cure out of care. The element is sin. The child with a bruised knee is a sinner, the woman cursing her abuser is a sinner, the man lamenting his failed vocation is a sinner, the youth stumbling over the hypocrisies

in society is a sinner. The condition that calls us into acts of caring dis-
arms us by its apparent innocence. The cry, the curse, the tears, the
confusion are uncalculated and undeserved. The urgency and innocence in the care-evoking condition obscures an element in the condition that we must not leave in obscurity, and that is this: We human
beings learn early and quickly to acquire expertise in using our
plight, whatever it is, to get those around us to do far more than getting us through or over the conditions; we learn how to use the condition of need as leverage in getting our own way—not our health, not
our maturity, not our peace, not justice, not our salvation, but our
way, our willful way.

This impulse to make oneself the center, to shrewdly or bullyingly
manipulate things and people to the service of self is what we, in our
theology textbooks at least, call sin. *Incurvatus se* was Augustine's
phrase for it, life curved in upon itself. We are created to open out
toward our neighbors, open upward toward God. We can only be
whole and healthy humans insofar as we do this. When we are in need,
when firsthand experience documents our inability to be whole beings
on our own, the first thing that can happen is that we become more
authentically human—need rips gashes in our self-containment and
opens us to the neighbor; a need blows holes in our roofed-in self-suffi-
ciency and opens us to God. But not necessarily, for the self-willed self
doesn't give up easily—it makes a persistent and determined stand to
use these need-generated openings as ways to pull God into *my* service, put the neighbors to *my* use. If unwary, the person providing care
is co-opted into feeding selfishness, which is to say, sin.

The only group of people in our society that shows any sign of
knowing this and acting on its knowledge is parents of young children.
Parents know that there is nothing less innocent than childhood. After
a few weeks, months at most, of responding unquestioningly to every
sign of need, mothers and fathers start getting smart, start filtering the
requests, cross-examining the wails. If they don't, they realize in a few
years and with a sense of dismay that it might be too late to do anything about it, that at the same time that they have been bandaging
knees, wiping away tears, buying designer jeans, running interference
for breakaway emotions that they have, at the same time, been feeding
pride, nourishing greed, fueling lust and cultivating envy.

But outside the circumstances of child raising, there doesn't
seem to be much awareness of this deviousness. The moment any one
of us says "Help me" and discovers how quickly others are suddenly

in attendance on us, making us the center, confirming our importance, a vast field for the exercise of sin—that is, getting our own god-
less and neighborless way—opens up. It is really quite incredible the
amount of illness, unhappiness, trouble, and pain that is actually chosen because it is such an effective way of being in control, of being
important, of exercising godlike prerogatives, of being recognized as
significant without entering the strenuous apprenticeship of becoming truly human, which always requires learning the love of God,
practicing love of neighbor.

And surely one reason that the awareness of this deviousness is
so dim among us is that as a wasteland society we do not take into
account this huge reality in the human condition, the sin.

Christians, perhaps, have less excuse than others in matters of
caring for being naive or ignorant about sin, for we go through life
with a book in our pocket or at least within reach that is both insistent
and convincing on the subject. But no one has much of an excuse—it
is, as Chesterton once pointed out, the only major Christian doctrine
that can be verified empirically.

But because of this, because of this refusal to take with full seriousness the nature and presence of sin, a great deal of caring becomes
a collaboration in selfishness, in self-pity, in self-destruction, in self-
indulgence—all the seemingly endless hyphenations that the self is
able to engineer. We wake up one morning and realize that we have
poured ourselves out in caring for these needy people and they aren't
getting any better. And we know that something is wrong in our caring; so we pray, "Teach us to care."

As pastors learn to care for persons in need what we mostly
learn is teach them to pray. This is our genius, this our central task.
This is why we are pastors. If we don't use the occasion of help as the
school for prayer, we abdicate our calling. Caring is a complex task.
No one person can do it all. An entire community is involved in care.
The pastor's task in the community of care is to teach the person in
need to pray—that is, to use this wound in the self that is closed in
upon itself as an opening through which we can listen to and answer
God. The wound is more than a wound—it is access to the outside, to
God, to others. Our primary task in exercising care is providing direction for a person in need to leave the small confines of the self-
defined world and enter the spaciousness of the God-defined world.

And I don't mean simply praying for them, although that is certainly part of it. I mean teaching them to pray, helping them to listen

to what God is saying, helping them to form an adequate response. Teaching people to pray is teaching them to use all the occasions of their lives as altars on which they receive God and his gifts. Teaching people to pray is teaching them that God is the one with whom they have to deal, not just ultimately and not just in general, but now and in detail. Teaching people to pray is not especially difficult work— any of us can do it using the Psalms and the Lord's Prayer as our texts—but it is difficult to stick with for we are constantly interrupted with urgent demands from family and friends to "do something." And it is difficult to get them to stick with us, for all the shortcut approaches for providing care, shortcutting God, promise far quicker results. And it is difficult to stick it out because, in the confusion and noise of wasteland traffic, it is hard to stay convinced that sin and God make much difference.

But difficult or not, it is our task—and nothing else is. If we do not keep to our assignment, we do not care. If we do not use the occasions of need to teach people to pray, we cave in to the proliferation of care in which there is no cure.

A single incident was revelatory for me in learning this essential component in prayer. Brenda was in the hospital and I went to see her. She was a social worker, mother of two daughters, wife, faithful in her worship. I had been her pastor for several years. I asked her what brought her to the hospital. She was in for tests—a lot of things didn't seem right in her body and her doctor couldn't figure out what was wrong. She would be there two or three days. We prayed together and I left. I came back in a couple of days and asked what the tests showed. Nothing much, she said. They want me to see a psychiatrist, they don't think it's physical, and I guess I think they are probably right. Knowing Brenda, I thought they were probably right too.

Following my usual script and given that cue I would ordinarily have said, "Would you like to talk about it?" Along with many pastors of my generation—this was the decade of the sixties—I was absorbed in psychology and counseling. I had received good training, found I had an aptitude for it, and loved the dynamics of the therapeutic encounter and conversation. And there was great need, for at the time there were virtually no counselors, psychological or psychiatric, in our community. Word of my availability got around. I was soon counseling not only my own parishioners but many of their friends as well. It was good work, and I found I liked being valued by the community in ways I never was as a mere pastor. But the work was also exhausting and at that moment beside Brenda's bed I didn't think I could handle one more set of complex emotions. I know she expected me to express my care for her by being her counselor. But at that moment I was just too tired, and I ducked. Instead of offering myself as a counselor to her, I used prayer as an escape exit and got out.

But I also began feeling guilty. I had let her down. I didn't care. After a couple of weeks my guilt got the better of my fatigue and I called her on the telephone, "Brenda, this is Pastor Peterson." We exchanged a few commonplaces, and then I said, "Is there anything I can do for you?" There was a fairly long pause that made me nervous, and then she said, "Yes, there is. I've been thinking a lot about this. Would you teach me to pray?"

That was the last thing I had expected from her. I had been a pastor for seven years and it was the first time anyone had asked me to teach them to pray. I had expected to do this and mostly this when I was ordained. But when no one seemed interested, at least not to the point of asking, I began responding to what they were asking. They were asking me to help them with their marriages, their kids, their emotions, their parents, and so I did. I was caring for them on the terms they set for me. God was not ignored in the work—I offered prayers for help and healing—but the problems of these people, the needs for which they requested my help, needs which I often helped them identify, were the agenda: need-oriented, problem-driven, solution-expectant. And I was usually able to work God into it somewhere or other. But more often than not, I was entering and accepting the world of the wasteland, a world where need, not God, was sovereign. I had become an unwitting collaborator in reinforcing their sin-self-centered worlds.

Brenda's request—"would you teach me to pray?"—returned me to my country of origin: God-oriented, mystery-attentive, obedience-ready. My central task among these people was not to help them solve their problems, but to help them see how their problems could help to solve them, serve as stimulus and goad to embrace the mystery of who they were as human beings, and then offer to be companion to them and teach them the language in this world in which we are God-created, Christ-invaded, Spirit-moved.

The prayer in our text is, "Teach us to care." Brenda's asking me to teach her to pray taught me to care. When care is restored to its true and proper context in the presence and action of God, becomes an aspect of prayer, it is at the same time removed from the controlling context of sin-twisted needs, self-serving ploys, the cultural/spiritual wasteland that Eliot described so well, the wasteland that drains all the cure out of care.

AND NOT TO CARE

The prayer, teach us to care, is balanced by the prayer, teach us not to care. In the business of caring there is something we need to learn how to do, but there is also something we need to learn not to do. And what we learn not to do is as important as what we learn to do.

A major contributing cause to the crisis in care is the widespread refusal to learn to not care, to accept limits, to respect boundaries. All through the traditions of caring there are frequent counsels to reticence, to detachment—holding back, letting go. But our times do not honor such counsel. We are hellbent on plowing full speed ahead, and damn the torpedoes. We are so sure that a little more knowledge will make us more effective, that a breakthrough in technology will usher in a new level of competence, that a larger budget will provide the resources for success, that to *not* do something when it is possible to do anything at all, is practically unthinkable.

The reason for the counsel to reticence is that the act of caring—responding to a person in need—takes place in an environment already surging with life, prodigal with energy, vitality, beauty. This life, creation in all its aspects, is complex, exceedingly complex, and far past the capacity of our understanding. We are far more ignorant of the world than we are knowledgeable of it. Despite our explorations and discoveries—all this information of what is before us, all this understanding of how it works—there is still far more that we don't know than what we do know. And, of all the parts of the creation that we come across in our travels, this part we call human is the most marvelous, most complex, most mysterious. We know a lot about bodies and minds and emotions and souls, about digestive systems, guilt and forgiveness, kidney functions, love and faith, moral strength, schizophrenia, growth hormones, growing in Christ, fetal development, character formation, synapses in the brain, and sin in the heart. But when we stand before a human being most of what is taking place is beyond us. And for that reason we had best not start poking around in what we don't understand lest we destroy something precious. There is much that is wrong with the world and the people in it, but there is far more that is right. Everything wrong takes place in an environment that is incredibly, dazzlingly alive, stunningly beautiful.

The pastor's primary assignment in the midst of this reality is to call men and women to worship. When we say "Let us worship God," as most of us do at least once a week, we stop everyone in their tracks, and shut them up for an hour or so. To my knowledge, no one has ever commented on the incalculable good that pastors do simply by getting hundreds of thousands of sinners off the streets for an hour a week and keeping them quiet. Gossip diminishes to a mere trickle, the crime rate plummets, there are fewer traffic accidents, air and water pollution decreases.

The single most obviously significant feature of worship is that we aren't doing anything. We aren't in charge. We aren't making anything happen. We are not exactly catatonic for we do go through a few motions—stand, kneel, sit, sing, offer, receive—but there is no usefulness to any of it. In the terminology of William James, these are acts that have no "cash value." Worship is mostly not-doing, not-saying. Implicit in the act of worship is this prayer, "Teach us . . . not to care."

We invite people into this time of not-doing, not-saying, not-caring regularly so that they can see what is going on, hear what is being said. The most important thing that is going on right now is what God is doing. The most important thing that is being said right now is what God is saying. Marvelous things being done. Amazing words being spoken. Look! Listen! Pastors are not the only ones calling attention to what is going on: poets help us listen, painters help us look. But pastors identify God in the action, God in the language.

What God has done and is doing is far more significant than anything you or anyone else will ever do. What God has spoken and is speaking is far more important than anything you or anyone else will ever say. But if we are not constantly brought to awareness of this huge God-dimension, trained in attentiveness to this immense God-presence, we will act and speak out of context, and if we act and speak out of context, no matter how well-intentioned we are, no matter how purely motivated we are, we will finally do far more damage than good.

We live on holy ground. We inhabit sacred space. This holy ground is subject to incredible violations. This sacred space suffers constant sacrilege. No matter—the holiness is there, the sacredness is there. If our lives, and in this case our caring, are shaped in response to the violations, to the sacrilege, and not out of the holy, they are shaped wrongly.

A number of years ago, my wife and three children were in Yellowstone National Park. It is the first of our wonderful national parks. I often think of our parks in relation to church sanctuaries. Just as the church sanctuary protects time and space for the contemplation of redemption, the wilderness sanctuary protects time and space for the contemplation of creation. Here is a place protected from exploitation where we can look at the earth "and the fullness thereof," be in adoration before the Creator and His creation. Yellowstone is the first of our national parks set apart for this purpose. I have always felt a personal involvement in the formation of this park because Cornelius Hedges, a Montana lawyer, was in on it. It was his idea. He got Teddy Roosevelt to come and see the country, camped with him on a little triangle of land between the Madison and Firehole Rivers, and convinced him of the importance of preserving wildness and naturalness against the exploitative trampling boots and bulldozers. As a schoolboy in Montana I attended Cornelius Hedges School. I took on the persona of Cornelius Hedges and took pride in his achievement in forming this creation sanctuary so that the real estate developers and amusement park operators didn't have a monopoly in defining valleys and lakes and trees.

So we were in a national park, as we often are while on vacation. Yellowstone. We were walking along a mountain meadow, profuse with wildflowers, when I saw a small child, five years old at most, thirty or forty yards away picking the wildflowers. He had a bouquet of fringed gentians in his fist, and was picking still more. It is against the law to pick wildflowers in the national parks. My children knew the Sierra Club text, "Take nothing but pictures, leave nothing but footprints" as well as they knew John 3:16. This is holy ground. This is a place to be in wonder. I was outraged that the sanctity of the ground was being violated. I yelled at the little boy, "Don't pick the flowers!" He looked at me, innocently wide-eyed—and now terrified. He dropped the flowers. Immediately my children were all over me, "Dad, you're worse than him, look how you scared him. That's terrible. You're awful!"

And they were right. You can't yell people into an awareness of holiness. You can't terrify people into the sacred. My indignant yelling was a far worse violation of the holy place than the boy picking a few fringed gentians. Later I reflected on how often I do this:

substitute bluster and yelling on behalf of God's holy presence instead of taking off my shoes and kneeling on the holy ground, and inviting anyone around to join me.

Plato contended that all authentic philosophy had its beginning in sense of wonder: existence is vastly beautiful, wonderfully good, majestically true—we can only get off on the right foot by beginning in adoration. All authentic *anything* has its beginning in a sense of wonder. All authentic caring begins in wonder, in adoration. If we don't begin in adoration we begin too small. If we begin by formulating a problem, by identifying a need, by tackling a necessary job, by launching a program, we reduce the reality that is before us to what we can do or get others to do. If we measure the world and the people in it according to our knowledge of it, we leave out most of the data, and the most significant data at that, the God data. How can we hope to do anything that is healing and whole and blessed if we are out of touch with our environment, unaware of the world?

And so in embarking on our tasks of caring for these troubled souls, sick bodies, disordered communities, we interrupt and say, "Let us worship God." Let us pay attention to the parts of the environment that we have ignored in our hurry in getting across the street while the light was still green. Let us pay attention to the eternal dimension in these people around us that we have missed in our determination to make them socially acceptable. "Lord, teach us not to care so we can see and hear what you and some others of your servants are doing in caring."

There are no holy places in the wasteland, no sacred space. There is no place for wonder. There is no awe. April, instead of being full of promise and bloom and fertility is "the cruellest month." In the wasteland anything you do is an improvement on what is there, so go ahead and do the best you can with what you have.

The metaphor of wasteland is replaced in Eliot's mature and praying poems (*The Four Quartets*) with a rose garden. The moment belief does its work, this so-called wasteland comes into focus as a rose garden—and in a rose garden you don't improve on what is there, you slow down, inhale deeply, take it in. You enter something that is more than you bring to it.

When we lose a sense of the holy, when there is no perception of the sacred, we will most certainly have a crisis in care. If we don't learn and practice the reverential reverence involved in not caring, we will destroy what we set out to honor.

And we pastors must take our share of responsibility in causing this crisis, for more often than not when people enter our churches on Sundays, we do not lead them in worship. We say "let us worship God," but then we go on to either divert them from the fullness of their lives by pepping them up with a show of pious cheerfulness, or we try to shake them out of what we perceive to be their directionless sloth by enlisting them in a task that will prove their moral worth.

Thousands and thousands of pastors have caved into the world's wasteland view of itself, and have gone to work, with the best will in the world but in the most appalling ignorance, to putting up billboards that advertise a God-product that will raise our standard of living, or organizing neighborhood groups to pick up the trash in the streets.

One of the exquisitely beautiful places in America is the Black Hills in South Dakota. But it is not easy to see the beauty. What you see mostly is garish and ugly signs, littering the landscape, inviting you to look at a freak, buy a trinket, sleep in expensive comfort. Instead of the wild beauty of the place being honored, it is exploited. And in the course of being exploited it is defaced. There are similarly beautiful places all over America that are similarly cheapened.

But what is far, far worse is the cheapening of our churches. A church is primarily a sanctuary—a definition through architecture of sacred space, a declaration that this ground is holy. A church sanctuary and the worship that takes place there is an invitation to enter into the essential holiness of all space and time, to get it right, to get it straight—to hear it said, and then to join in the saying, "Holy, holy, holy. Lord God Almighty, heaven and earth are full of your glory." But more often than not, the people who approach these places set apart to ponder and realize the beauty of holiness are hustled and recruited— diverted from the unhappy conditions in which they live, enlisted in some program that will give them weekend relief from the boredom of their ordinary life. Sadly, the hustlers and recruiters are mostly the pastors. It is all done in the name of Jesus, of course, but the name Jesus functions as the Black Hills do, as pretext and occasion for the entrepreneurial spirit. Sanctuaries are cluttered with signs and posters of what people are doing or could be doing and interfering with and obscuring the holy—God present in creation and salvation, God become flesh and dwelling among us, God making the world and resting, God roaring in the thunder, whispering in the still small voice, God on the cross, God in the bread and wine. God. Holy, Holy, Holy.

What kind of world is this in which we care? As we go about our work, to what do we give witness? Is it "holy, holy, holy" or

In this decayed hole among the mountains
In the faint moonlight, the grass is singing
Over the tumbled graves, about the chapel
There is the empty chapel, only the wind's home.
                    (*The Wasteland*, lines 386–389)

I don't say that this is easy, only that it is necessary, clearing the clutter so that the space we work in can be perceived as holy. Quieting the noise so that the time we live in can be perceived as sacred. Otherwise we become collaborators in the mess-making and noise-making that have so deeply penetrated the vocations of caregiving.

*   *   *

Teach us to care: teach us to use all these occasions of need that are the agenda of our work as access to God, access to neighbor; teach us to care by teaching to pray so that human need becomes occasion for entering into and embracing the presence and action of God in this life; teach us to care by teaching to pray so that those with whom we work are not less human through our caring but more human; teach us to care so that we do not become collaborators in self-centeredness but rather companions in God-exploration; teach us to use each act of caring as an act of praying so that this person in the act of being cared for experiences dignity instead of condescension, realizes the glory of being in on the salvation and blessing and healing of God and is not driven further into neurosis and the wasteland of self.

And not to care: teach us to be reverential in all these occasions of need that are the agenda of our work, aware that you were "long beforehand" with this person, creating and loving, saving and wooing; teach us the humility of not-caring so that we do not use anyone's need as a workshop to cobble together makeshift messianic work that inflates our importance and indispensability; teach us to be in wonder and adoration before the beauties of creation and the glories of salvation, especially as they come to us in these humans who have come to think of themselves as violated and degraded and rejected; teach us the reticence of restraint of not-caring so that in our eagerness to do good we do not ignorantly interfere in your caring; teach us not to care so that we have time and energy and space to realize that all our work is done on holy ground in your holy name, that people and communities in need are not a wasteland where we feverishly and faithlessly set up shop but a garden in which we work contemplatively.

Suffer us not to mock ourselves with falsehood
Teach us to care, and not to care.
Teach us to sit still.
Even among these rocks.
                    (*Ash Wednesday*)

NARRATIVE:

No Safe Conduct

WILLIAM VISICK

I am a forty-eight year old physician who has been practicing anesthesi-ology for twenty years. Two years ago I had a bout with the flu. It was one of those years when everyone's symptoms seemed to last for weeks instead of days. Slowly, I began to get over it, but the headaches stayed on, and in some ways, even seemed to get worse. They bothered me more when I leaned over, and my head felt continually "stuffed up."

I began to think, "Something is wrong inside my head." But I could not imagine what that might be. I considered scheduling an MRI scan. With the intention of doing things "the right way," I called the appropriate doctor and said, "I've had headaches for a month. This is very unusual for me. I'm thinking of scheduling a scan. What do you think?" He replied, "Oh, there are lots of reasons for headaches. Don't do that. Come into my office and see me." "Okay," I said. "How about this afternoon?" "I have space a week from Friday," he said. "Sign me up," I responded, thinking, "I can't wait that long, something is WRONG here!"

I walked straight to the MRI lab and scheduled a scan to follow my last case the next day. By the end of the next day I knew I had a brain tumor. A day and a half later, I was a patient under the knife.

It was a bad one. Glioblastoma Multiforme, the same kind of brain tumor that felled Lee Atwater the previous year. I knew what it meant. I am a doctor. Doctors know that gliomas of the brain, oat cell carcinomas of the lung, and melanomas are fatal. I thought the end was imminent. I was in despair. I had two strapping, full of life teenage sons. I loved my wife. I was a good doctor. I was a more than decent person. People depended on me. I had struggled to get where I was. I didn't

---

[EDITOR'S NOTE: Dr. William Visick died in his home on June 9, 1992.]

smoke. I didn't eat bacon with nitrites. I had a lot to see, do, and enjoy yet.

And I was terrified. I did not know how to do this. I have seen patients die. I have been there when the life went out. But, me! I do not know how to do this! I'm not ready. Who will help me understand what is happening? Who will be with me along the way? Where am I going?

I looked for hope, and I looked for help. "What are my chances?" I asked the radiation oncologist. "You have the best constellation of features for this cell type," he said. "A thirty percent chance of surviving three years." Some, but small hope. My doctor's realism and my personality checked too much hope or too much denial of the facts. I stoically pushed ahead with the radiation treatments and through unexpected side effects and complications: erytheme multiforme (a skin reaction like a burn), cerebritis (worse headaches than before), more months in the hospital, and recovery time at home during which I had to relearn some of the most elementary and primitive aspects of living.

Sometimes the professional helpers missed the mark and helped not at all: The internationally famous urologist and endocrinologist who seemed simply to plug a list of symptoms into a standardized decision tree, ordered some tests, and never called back. A familiar occurrence in medicine.

Sometimes the professionals hit the mark square in the center: The family doctor who listened carefully and said, "That reminds me of recovering victims of the concentration camps. This is what helped them. Let's try it." The oncologist who told me about a lady lawyer from Denver who had the same constellation of findings two years ago and now is back at work. When the monthly CAT scans continued to look better, the oncologist, rejoicing with me, identified with me, saying, "Remember, your CAT scan is *my* CAT scan. This could be me!"

Several other people were supportive and healing. One of the OR nurses became the Hound of Heaven. Every morning after my radiation treatments at the University of California Medical Center, I returned to my car to find she had left a cheerful note saying, "Keep on!," or some cookies, or a card.

When I was afraid to go to sleep at night, or I could not, my friends came over and massaged my feet until I did. A doctor friend gave me a whimsical, colorful Bula hat to cover my bald head. A friend gave me a tape of Kiri Te Kanawa singing Gounod's *Sanctus*. I played it over and over and was immersed in beauty and impelled to feel there is something bigger than me and my horrible circumstances.

My therapist listens. He helps me begin to understand that, first, there is *no safe conduct*, and, second, I am going through what we all go through at some time. We *all* will die; I may just be finding myself here sooner than usual. He let me know that he cares, that he "regards" me.

I know that I am loved. I know that I am not alone. Gradually, I began to feel better, became stronger. The follow-up CAT scans continue unremarkable after two years, and I can smile and nod at the guy in the town square who wears the t-shirt that reads, "Eat well, stay fit, die anyway."

The Caring Physician: Balancing the Three Es: Effectiveness, Efficiency, and Empathy

E. Dawn Swaby-Ellis

I am deeply honored to have been asked to consider the crisis of care in the helping professions. In sharing with one of my colleagues my trepidation about contributing to a book along with such distinguished scholars as Robert Bellah, Charles Taylor, Patricia Benner, and other celebrated authors, I was encouraged when he said, "You're one of the few people who can really tell it like it is from your day-to-day experience—give the view from the trenches, so to speak!"

Being in the trenches for me is practicing and teaching pediatrics at Grady Hospital in downtown Atlanta, one of the largest public hospitals in the nation. Since 1892, Grady, like all large public hospitals, has existed primarily to treat the indigent sick and provide medical assistance during emergencies. Fifty-thousand patients are admitted each year to the 900-bed facility, and there are 850,000 outpatient visits. To many of the 70,000 children who visit the pediatrics emergency room each year, Grady is their primary care doctor. In typical public hospital tradition, Grady is also a major site for the training of the medical students of Emory and Morehouse Universities.

For the past five years, I have worn many hats. My main responsibilities have been to direct the third-year clerkship for medical students in pediatrics and the medical care of neonatal intensive care graduates in the outpatient follow-up clinic. Until recently, finding a replacement person for either of these activities has been like pulling the teeth of an elephant.

The reality of my life at Grady is illustrated by the events of the morning on which I tried to complete this manuscript. As I sat down to weave the threads of my thoughts together, I felt relieved that a neonatologist interested in developmental follow-up was scheduled to be in the clinic within a few hours. My work was interrupted, however, by an anxious telephone call from one of my team workers, the nurse practitioner who directs the follow-up clinic: "Dawn, there is a sick child here who needs to be seen by a physician." My stress level instantly rose, my gastric juices poured, and my voice became terse, but my response was immediate: "I'll be there in a minute." On my way over to the clinic, I prayed for a peaceful spirit and struggled to transform my resentment over the interruption into the will to care for this child: "Lord, help me to believe in your ability to provide care through me. Help me to believe that all things work together for good to those who love you and are called to your purpose. Give me your priorities for today. Give me wisdom in dealing with this child."

Although the scenario changes, I face this same dilemma daily in my life: I am trying to write a paper, but a sick child needs my help; I need to finish making a diagnosis, but a medical student arrives unannounced with a crisis; I am looking forward to discussing my day with a friend, but my four-year-old son desperately wants me to admire his latest Lego creation. Whatever the competing factions, my challenge is the same: to be effective, efficient, and empathic. For physicians in the United States, the difficulty of balancing these responsibilities has limited our ability to care and led to a crisis in our delivery of care. A recent American Medical Society survey indicates that less than half of the American public believes that "doctors usually explain things well to their patients," three fourths think that "doctors keep patients waiting too long," two thirds think that "doctors are too interested in making money," and six out of ten believe that "doctors don't care about people as much as they used to" (Harvey, Lynn K. and S. C. Shubat, *Physician Opinion on Health Care Issues*, Chicago: American Medical Association, May, 1992, pp. i–ii, 25–26). Public dissatisfaction with doctors is reflected in the growth of the self-care and wellness industries as well as in the rise of the number of malpractice suits.

The public perception of noncaring physicians is accompanied by evidence that, despite a greater expenditure on health care than other countries, the American health care system is failing its most vulnerable citizens. Because a fifth of the nation's children live in poverty, the health of American children is particularly at risk. Many of the nation's poor do not qualify for Medicaid and Medicare, and many physicians do not accept patients on these health plans. A recent conference sponsored by the American Academy of Pediatrics, the National Commission to Prevent Infant Mortality, the National Commission on Children, and the House Select Committee on Children, Youth, and Families compared the health of children in the

United States with those in Canada, France, Great Britain, the Netherlands, Norway, and Sweden (*Pediatrics*, 86 (6), Dec., 1990, pt. 2, supplement, pp. 1025–1027). The statistics showed that:

- American childhood injury mortality rates are greater than those in every comparison country;
- Immunization against diphtheria and tetanus averages 41 percent higher in Europe than in the United States;
- America ranks 16th in the world in postneonatal mortality; and
- The pregnancy rate for American adolescents is twice that of Great Britain, triple that of Sweden, and seven times that of the Netherlands.

The rate of American infant mortality is so high in comparison to other countries that the conference did not even compare those statistics.

It is disturbing that the crisis in our delivery of medical care should occur at the close of a century that has witnessed the most rapid development in life-sustaining technology of any other time. What has been lost as physicians have moved from their role of medicine man, wound healer, barber surgeon, minister, and family physician to diagnostician, scientist, technological expert, and life saver? To help answer this question, I asked several colleagues for their assessment of the problem. All of them perceived themselves as caring physicians, but they were frustrated by a health care system that discourages the development of a close relationship between doctor and patient.

Dr. *A*, a specialist at a public hospital, believes that "continuity of care is essential for the ideal caring practice of medicine." Although continuity of care is difficult to provide in private practice and impossible to achieve in the hospital emergency room, Dr. *A* argues that, to solve the current crisis of care, we must:

> move back to more continuous relationships with patients, really having knowledge of them, as opposed to an assembly line practice of medicine, where we give only episodic care. We should focus on the doctor-patient relationship more. When this is sacrificed for convenience, economics, or efficiency, we sacrifice our capacity to care.

There are inherent contradictions in our practice of medicine in a society in which money is the measure of worth. A quick, efficient encounter with a patient may cost less, but is it better than a longer, more time-consuming one? Society must choose what it values most: economy or empathy.

A generalist at a public hospital, Dr. B believes that physicians' ability to care is limited by a health care system that demands quantity rather than quality of care:

> Our ability to care is a function of the numbers of patients we have to see. In the past, doctors were more involved with entire families and knew their patients both medically and socially. Now, we often share our responsibilities with other doctors, which interrupts the continuity of care that we're able to provide. Care seems to be less personal. I think we adopt a less caring attitude as a means of self-protection while we focus on seeing more and more patients during a day.
>
> Some, though not all, clerks and receptionists in hospitals and doctors' offices view their work as just a job. They often do not understand that, to do their job well, they must be devoted to their patients' concerns. As a woman with a family, I understand the demands on staff time, but potential employees need to be screened for their willingness to listen and place themselves in their patients' shoes. The solution lies with the creation of a caring atmosphere in which doctors, nurses, technicians, physical therapists, and medical personnel combine their efforts to care for their patients.

Dr. B admits that patients' eagerness to bring malpractice suits may discourage doctors from forming a personal relationship with them, but she views such litigious attitudes as a response to, rather than a cause of, the impersonality of many doctor/patient interactions:

> There have been changes on the patient's side of things, too. Patients are more informed, more critical, more judgmental, and, yes, more litigious, [but] the higher frequency of liability issues relates to the loss of the personal relationship between doctor and patient.

Dr. C, a specialist who works in a university-hospital setting, echoes many physicians' frustration with the American health care system, which he believes does not equitably provide treatment and hospitalization for all citizens:

> The chief obstacle to my being able to provide effective care is [a] system of health care that is inadequate for the patient's needs . . . and forces the physician to waste enormous amounts of time trying to find ways around the obstacles set up to discourage proper care. Persuading and cajoling people to provide drugs and other services to poor patients is an inefficient use of physicians' time and erodes our sense of achievement as doctors.

According to Dr. C, physicians could provide better care to their patients under a health care system that "provided the same level of services, with the same expertise to all patients" regardless of their income, location, or personal characteristics.

Even though Dr. D's interaction with patients is limited to the time they spend in intensive care, she has learned to develop and maintain rapport with them and their families, which she believes is especially important when the diagnosis is discouraging or unclear:

> To teach this point to residents and fellows, I use a film called "The Other End of the Endotracheal Tube." It's about a physician who received good care in the intensive unit, saw all his lines placed and his vital organs monitored, but was not talked to by any of his physician colleagues. Consequently, he felt uncared for and alone a lot, especially when his condition worsened and he could not find anyone who wanted to talk about death. I talk to families more frequently when their child is very sick and less frequently when the child is getting better. Some people think it should be the reverse, but when the patient is sickest, the family needs the most contact with the physician.

Being a patient herself helped Dr. D develop a caring practice. When her knee was injured, she chose a physician who not only was an expert at fixing knees but could also support her emotionally in case the operation was not successful. Dr. D believes that a physician's ability to *care* can often be more important than his or her ability to *cure*:

I think caring is a motivational concept; it's not externally seen, but it can be recognized by other co-workers, nursing staff, and patients. I have a stronger motivation to care now than I did as a medical student when . . . I saw medical practice as curing disease rather than as a process of alleviating suffering. . . . Now I'm more concerned with making sure that science is integrated into practice and made palatable to the patient.

My colleagues agreed that the crisis of care in the medical profession will escalate unless American policymakers and medical professionals join forces to advocate the following steps:

- Adoption of a universal health care policy that provides for the basic health care needs of every citizen;
- Distribution of hospital and clinic services in an equitable manner;
- Control of the development of medical technology to balance the need for new services with our ability to deliver optimum care to all;
- Limitation of unnecessary medical investigation; and
- Expansion of the medical school curriculum to emphasize, in addition to the knowledge and management of disease, the development of
  1. good communication skills,
  2. effective interviewing techniques,
  3. cultural sensitivity,
  4. tools for teaching health maintenance and illness prevention, and
  5. methods for determining the appropriate use of technology.

Finding the will to take these steps depends on America's ability to transform the philosophy of individualism on which our society is based into one that values the interdependence of all citizens. At the conference on child health I mentioned earlier, Birt Harvey noted that "[w]e have always considered individualism our ideal, and the concept is rooted firmly in our frontier spirit and our system of free enterprise" ("Epilogue," in *Child Health in 1990: The United States Compared to Canada, England, and Wales, France, The Netherlands, and Norway*, Proceedings of a Conference on Cross-National Comparisons of Child

Health, *Pediatrics*, 86(6), Dec. 1990, supplement, p. 1127). This empha-
sizes the welfare of the individual over that of the group. European
thought is oriented more toward interdependence, with greater
emphasis on the well-being of the group. Harvey writes, "What we
really must do is change our philosophy regarding children" (p. 1026).

Finding a solution to the crisis of *caring* in the medical profession is more complicated and involves some self-examination. The
complexity of the problem was brought home to me one day many
years ago while I cared for patients as a weekly volunteer at a church-
based health clinic in Kingston, Jamaica. It had been a long day, and I
was physically and emotionally tired. I wondered why I had agreed
to my friend (Dr. Tony Allen's) request that I work in this clinic,
which serves people who cannot afford health care in the city. After
all, my days were filled with caring for patients at the University hospital where I worked. Besides, the clinic had not even started to serve
children, and I hated seeing "little old ladies," whose vague pains
never seemed to have any anatomical source.

As I sat in my chair waiting for the first patient to arrive, I prayed
that God would let me know whether He wanted me to continue to
work in the clinic. An elderly woman limped into the examination
room, sat gingerly down, and started reciting a litany of complaints:
pain in her hip, knee, and back; tightness in her neck; shivers running
down her spine; cold sweats. "Well, here we go again," I thought as I
began a thorough examination. "It could be a pinched nerve or arthri-
tis. After all, she's in her late sixties." Suddenly, I was conscious of a
voice in my ear, "But, Dawn, do you *love* her?" I was used to hearing
the voice of the Holy Spirit by now, and I knew that He spoke in all
sorts of ways. I needed to hear it again. "But, do you *love* her?"

For a moment, I was speechless. Then I remembered my patient
saying something about her son in the initial interview, and I said,
"Tell me about your son." The woman's face became animated, and
she talked for the next fifteen minutes about her son, his staying out
late at night, his failure to keep a job, his getting into bad company. I
began to feel a real interest in this woman and her life. Although I
didn't know what to do, I offered to pray with her for her son. One
advantage of this clinic was that prayer with patients was encouraged. On her next visit two weeks later, I asked her about her limp. At
first, she looked puzzled. Then she smiled, and a radiance lit up her
face, "Oh, doctor," she said. "Don't worry about my hip. Let me tell
you about my son! He's staying home now, he got a job, and he don't

keep that company any more. I'm so happy! Thank you for your prayers. I'm so glad I came to this clinic!"

This type of miraculous experience does not occur daily in my practice, but God gave me insight into the significance of caring that day. I learned that caring for patients comes out of true concern and love for them. In the case of this woman, caring gave me the power to listen and recall the really important concerns on her heart. If I had merely focused on curing her symptoms, our interaction may not have had any beneficial effect.

From ancient times to the present, master physicians have always understood the relationship between caring and curing. As early as the fourth century B.C., the writings of the Greek physician Hippocrates contain the following precept: "For where the love of man is, there is also the love of the art [of medicine]" (*Precepts*, 6). Although not all of these writings are attributed to Hippocrates himself, he clearly placed accurate observation of the patient at the center of his practice and emphasized that cure is dependent on the physician's view of the patient. During the second century A.D., the Chinese physician Chang Chung Kin also advocated the study of diseases based on close observation of the patient. Maimonides, a Jewish physician in the twelfth century, is known for approaching his patients as human beings rather than case studies. Other physicians with reputations for being caring and observant include Drs. Thomas Browne, Peter Lowe, William Osler, Benjamin Rush, and Thomas Syndenham.

Great medical scientists and clinicians have consistently sought to return the patient to center stage and called for the humane practice of medicine to the poor. During the early part of the twentieth century, Dr. Francis Peabody continued in this tradition, writing in *The Care of the Patient* (JAMA 88:887–892, 1927): "One of the essential qualities of the clinician is an interest in humanity, for the secret of care *of* the patient is caring *for* the patient." (Emphasis added.)

I believe that physicians' ability to care depends on the following factors:

- Their character;
- The quality of interaction they shared with their primary caregivers;
- Their life experiences and stage of growth;
- Their motivation to become a physician (*e.g.*, to serve, to care, to cure, to comfort, to educate, to empower, to investigate, or to achieve status, power, privilege, and respect);

- Their view of the medical profession (*e.g.*, as work, a career, a vocation, or a calling);
- The view of their family, friends, colleagues, and faith tradition toward their decision to practice medicine;
- Their clinical method; and
- The socio-political influences on them and their patients.

My own journey in learning how to care began in a family whose values were based on a strong Christian faith and belief in the innate worth of every human being. The products of an African slave, a European slavemaster, and Indian indentured laborers, my parents taught me the importance of shaping my mind through higher education, respecting my elders' wisdom and experience, understanding my heritage, accepting responsibility for my actions, and striving for excellence in all that I do.

When I announced at age fifteen that I wanted to be a doctor, my mother, a nurse, was delighted despite her friends' fears that I would be less feminine and never find a husband. After watching me help my pets give birth, she knew I had the aptitude to be either a doctor or a veterinarian. Although my father seemed pleased about my decision, he went to great lengths to explain how hard the training would be, the gory sights I would see, and the sleepless nights I would have. He suggested and probably arranged that I spend several summers working in the pathology department of the nearby university under the supervision of his good friend, a professor of pathology.

As a morbid anatomy technician, I had responsibility for processing and filing surgical and postmortem material. This was the lowest job on the totem pole of histopathological technicians, but whenever I made a labeling mistake, the professor called me into his office for a stern lecture on the dire consequences of my error: the possibility that a wrong diagnosis would be ascribed to a patient, whose liver or breast might then be mistakenly removed. His excessive reaction was undoubtedly the collaborative work of my father and his friend to ensure that I would have no romantic illusions about the life of a doctor.

During my training in medical school, my professors and mentors did much to shape my character as a caring physician. As an intern, I remember working with a neurosurgeon who not only performed craniotomies but knew all his patients by name, taking careful note of their profession or trade so that he could talk to them after surgery about how the results would affect their lives. One of my professors of medicine always knew more of his patients' history than the intern, resident, and student put together. His secret, we later discovered, was to return to the wards in the evening, sit beside the patients' beds, and let them talk about their illness. "Seventy-five percent of your diagnosis," he would tell us, "should be based on the narrative that the patient relates about the illness. Twenty percent should come after the physical. The laboratory should confirm your suspicions, and the remaining five percent may come after perusing the literature and discussing the patient with other colleagues."

My first professor of pediatrics taught me to believe in my own power to diagnose, based on reason and experience. From him, I learned to have the courage of my convictions, even if the senior resident disagreed with me. I was also impressed by the head of my department, who rushed to the hospital to comfort the grieving mother of a child I was caring for that had suddenly died on Christmas Eve. I watched as he put his arms around her and allowed her to sob until there were no more tears. Then he found me, a young intern, in tears in a side hall and comforted me by calming my fears that something could have been done to save the child. Later, he discussed the postmortem findings with me, which revealed a rare occurrence of pulmonary embolism in a healthy child who had been hospitalized for Stevens-Johnson's syndrome.

These physicians all followed the Flexner biomedical model, named after Abraham Flexner, whose 1910 report to the Carnegie Foundation placed American medical education on a firm scientific foundation. At a recent conference on teaching medical interviewing organized by the Task Force on Physician and Patient, now The American Academy on Physician and Patient, I was exposed to the biopsychosocial model proposed by George Engel. Never since the beginning of my training have I attended a conference that focused on physicians' interaction with patients, and I came away from it validated in the depths of my being. The biopsychosocial model expands our understanding of the causes of disease to encompass the psychological, social, and cultural determinants. (See Engel, "The Need for a New Medical Model: A Challenge for Biomedicine," *Science* 196:129–136 1977). Because this model relies on an analysis of how patients communicate the symptoms of disease, physicians that follow it will need more training in medical interviewing, psychology, sociology, and anthropology than students currently receive in medical school.

Paul Tournier, the Swiss physician and psychologist who introduced me to the link between mental and physical health, expands the biopsychosocial model to include a spiritual dimension. His book, *The Doctor's Casebook in the Light of the Bible* (tr. Edwin Hudson, London: SCM Press, NY: Harper, 1960), describes the connection between patients' symptoms and their relationship with God. In an interview with a patient who had chronic recurrent unexplained symptoms, Tournier was able to uncover suppressed guilt about an immoral relationship and pain about never being loved by a parent. Using the power of confession and self-understanding, Tournier helped the patient restore her relationship with a loved one, which led to the healing of her physical complaint.

My greatest teacher in learning how to care has been the Holy Spirit. It is one thing to be a Christian who wishes to live a life of obedience to God by showing love to mankind. It is another thing to integrate our faith into the fabric of our being so that our actions mirror our spiritual beliefs. Learning to be really concerned for our patients' welfare, to view things from their perspective, to show empathy, and to enter into their grief is a continuous lesson. I think of the words of Jesus Christ in Matthew 25:42-43 as I walk down Butler Street in Atlanta daily, trying to avoid the drunks and paranoid homeless who cross my path toward the entrance to Grady Hospital: "When you saw me hungry, sick, and in prison, did you care for me?" Our challenge is to love and care for each and every human being, as Jesus did. Mother Theresa ascribes her concern for the untouchables of Delhi as a function of her love and obedience to Jesus Christ. Being the representatives of Jesus in our world is an awesome challenge, but we must have the courage to act as agents for change.

Since I came to America from Jamaica nine years ago, I have had the privilege of working with many groups made up of caring health professionals. The Christian Community Health Fellowship shows its concern for the health care of the poor in rural and urban areas across the nation. The Carter Center in Atlanta provides leadership and resources to improve the health of children in the Third World. Christ House provides a ministry to the homeless in Washington, D.C. All of these groups are run by people who care more for others than for their personal advancement and comfort. I am excited about the possibility of a reawakening of that vision in churches all over America. The Church can become the center for physical as well as spiritual healing. As the writer of Proverbs 18:14 reminds us, "The human spirit will endure sickness, but a broken spirit, who can bear?" Perhaps it is time for physicians to acknowledge their limitations and form partnerships with churches to serve the people.

Balancing the responsibilities of effectiveness, efficiency, and empathy will never be an easy task. Our choices may be simplified, however, if we always seek to place our patients first. If we listen to our patients, we will be able to enter into a dialogue with them. If we try to communicate with our patients, we will recognize the importance of educating them. If we search for solutions to their problems, we will be able to understand and empathize with them. If we recognize our own limitations, we will reach out for help from our colleagues and from God, who alone can heal the body and change the human heart. The measurement of our effectiveness in His eyes will come at the end of our journey when we hear His voice: "Well done, my good and faithful servant! Enter now into the joy of your Lord" (Matthew 25:23).

NARRATIVE:

To Care Is to Listen

MIMA BAIRD

In our chosen profession as psychotherapists, we care for and about people. We very consciously and continuously care, hour by hour and client by client. The extension and embodiment of our caring is the quality of our listening. It is not a static skill or level of competence that is achieved once and for all, but a dynamic and constantly changing awareness that we have to fine-tune and focus with each individual in every hour.

It takes discipline and commitment to reach into ourselves to that quiet, calm place deep within, where we leave the familiar structure of diagnoses, interpretations, and schedules to shift to that focused attention that creates an oasis, a haven, a strong, solid place that is not threatened by the reverberations of anger, a place where the timid and frightened whisper of a wounded and unheard soul can be heard. Our desire and ability to hear invites the other to listen, to hear, and to respect his or her own story and process.

In the past few years I have been privileged to be taught by our grandchildren. The lessons are often simple, profound, and go to the heart of matters in ways that textbooks never can. At a gathering of the clan, a little handpainted red chair from Mexico caught the eye and desire of the four-year-old and his two-and-a-half-year-old cousin. Adults used the situation as an opportunity for the children to learn about sharing and taking turns. The attention shifted back to the flow of adult conversation until a screech drew everyone's attention to a heated battle being fought over the little red chair.

As fathers and mothers, aunts and uncles intervened scolding the four-year-old for not being willing to share, the usually mellow child began to escalate until he was beyond words. Finally someone wondered whether his momentarily leaving the chair was not an indication that his turn was finished, but rather that he had wanted to get his bear and finish his turn in the chair. This had been seen by his two-and-a-half-year-old cousin as a signal to take immediate possession of the chair.

As soon as someone accurately "heard" and understood the context of the scenario, calm returned, turns were once again negotiated,
and both children enjoyed the chair for the rest of their interest span.
How often do our clients, or we ourselves, begin to escalate until someone cares enough to listen and our actions are understood?

As a psychotherapist, I have been privileged to see the enlivening
and healing process happen before my eyes as individuals have been
able to hear their lives without distortion or judgment. I know, both theoretically and experientially, the powerful impact of being heard by
another and by one's self. A brief recent experience of mine reminded
me once again of the healing effect of being cared for by being heard
accurately.

In the midst of an unusually busy schedule, a routine yearly physical exam revealed something suspicious that the surgeon wanted to
biopsy. To protect my family from unnecessary worry until all the facts
were in hand, and to be sure that I did not "leak" any of my personal
process into therapy hours (especially with several clients who were in
the midst of grieving cancer-related deaths), I very consciously decided
to play it "cool," casually mentioning to my family that I would be
going to the hospital on Friday for some tests.

I must have mentioned it so casually that the remark just slid by
and no one appeared to hear it. By playing it cool, I was also building a
seawall against the rising tide of anxiety and fear that felt like it could
sweep me off my feet. I had celebrated passing the five-year mark after
cancer surgery, and I was not prepared to walk that path again.

On Thursday I had an appointment with my therapist and used
the hour for consultation on a difficult case. Only toward the end of the
hour did I mention that I was going to have a biopsy the next day and
talked briefly about the procedure, the inconvenience of having to rear-
range my schedule, and so on. This very traditionally trained psychiatrist said something he had never said before, "Feel free to call me
anytime after the procedure if you'd like to talk." I burst into tears that
welled up from that part of me that I had been isolating and not hearing.

To experience being truly heard was to experience compassion
and concern for my whole self. It was a quality of care that then freed
me to comfort and tend to that part of myself that had been silenced,
the part that I had shut up and shut off. It was with a sense of relief and
gratitude that I left the message that the biopsy results were negative. I
was grateful that I had been heard. To care is to listen; to hear is to care.

Preparing Students for the World

JAIME ESCALANTE

What makes a teacher a good teacher? A teacher must have self-respect. A teacher with self-respect will be personally confident and hopeful about the future. A teacher with positive feelings about him or herself will be able to have such feelings about the students. Teachers must be in charge of their own lives and able to accept responsibility for their failures. Good teachers look, act, and talk energetically and with enthusiasm every day. They must have the energy of the hottest volcano. Knowledge of the subject is essential in good teaching, as is the ability to have good relationships with the students, motivate them, and talk to them one-on-one as human beings. A teacher needs the memory of an elephant, the precision of a calculator, the understanding of a doctor with a patient in pain, the patience of a turtle trying to cross the street at rush hour, and the tenacity of a spider carefully weaving its web. With the right desire and commitment to teaching, anybody can do it.

What we do in our classrooms will be reflected in our society. We teachers must draw out the potential in our students. I love teaching in the classroom and lighting the fire of mathematics in the hearts of my students. I love to spark the idea of education in their minds. That is what a teacher should be doing in whatever subject that teacher teaches. The skills and expertise of a nation's work force are the foundation of the nation's economic success. Right now in this country that foundation is weak. High schools are not producing students to stand and deliver in the face of the challenge of the twenty-first century.

Youngsters face significant turning points in their lives. They have the chance to better their lives and contribute to their country by taking advantage of the opportunities offered in their schools. The ages ten through fifteen years are critical. With the beginning of puberty, children develop rapidly, more rapidly than during the previous five years. This time of rapid development offers teachers the opportunity to take advantage of the potential these kids bring to the school and to the classroom. Society will benefit from that potential if it is developed. Unfortunately, many kids in this age group are at risk for many problems, and we may not reach them in time.

Many kids become sexually active in adolescence and some become pregnant. As high school teachers we face these complications in our students' lives, as well as their exposure to gangs, drugs, AIDS, and so on. We must recognize the common denominator in these problems: the fundamental breakdown in the human relationship between parents and child. It is essential that a good relationship exist between the parents and the child, and we teachers need to keep that in mind. It is also essential that there be a good relationship between the teacher and the student. It takes parents and teachers together to change the crisis of care that affects the young people in our country.

In my high school, I invite the parents to visit my classroom. I say to the parents, "Look, I want to give you some advice. I need you to want to do the following: Every time you talk to your kid, talk with love. Love without limits, unconditional love. Don't tell your kid, 'If you do this, if you do that, you're going to get this.' No. Remember that kid belongs to you. That kid does not belong to the park or the street or the school. That kid is your responsibility. Second, I'm going to ask you this: every time you discipline your kid, you must also show love. Love motivates discipline. This is how your kid is going to learn responsibility. The third piece of advice is, maybe, the most difficult: you must understand your teenager. You and I will work on this together. Together we're going to work to help this child reach the highest positive degree of personal development. I need your help. School alone cannot educate. Fourth, every time your child talks to you, wake up. An opportunity is knocking on your door. The last favor I'm going to ask you as a parent is that you listen when your child approaches you and talks to you. Be interested. Don't put your child down; don't be shocked; don't laugh; don't talk about your own problems. Help your child find his or her own solutions. This is your assignment. If you do these things I ask, you will create an environment of love and learning for your child, and you will be giving your country a better tomorrow."

When students walk into my classroom, they see posters of famous athletes decorating the walls. Those are a principal part of my teaching. I have Wilt Chamberlain, Jerry West, and many others. During the first week of class I talk about Wilt Chamberlain. I say to my students, "You know what? This guy used to pull lots of rebounds, used to block a great number of shots. The relationship between our classroom team and the Lakers is simple: don't let any homework assignment block you; don't be intimidated by words like 'calculus' and 'algebra.' You're the best. You can do it. Anybody could do it. All I need from you is *ganas* which translated into English means 'desire,' 'desire to learn.'"

The next week I talk about my favorite player, the famous number 44, Jerry West. I say to my students, "You know, they used to call him 'Mr. Clutch.' Why? Because when the team needed a point during the last seconds of the game, they'd throw the ball to him knowing he would come through for them. That's why they called him 'Mr. Clutch'! And I expect the same reflexes from you. When I ask you a question, I expect the correct answer. When I expect that, you can do it. The only thing I need from you is *ganas*."

I tell my students that one day I spoke with Jerry West. I asked him why his friends called him "Mr. Clutch." He said,"Because even though I don't have a game in my schedule, I take the ball out and shoot the basketball at least five hundred times." I tell my students, "That's why Jerry West was a skillful shooter. I'm asking the same thing of you. Are you filled with the instructions from your teacher and from your mom and dad? Tomorrow or another day when you go to college, you must not sit in the back. Sit in the front. People are watching you. They think you cannot do it. I know you can do it, and that's a big plus to your name."

With my students I also post formulas. Under the clock I have a formula that reads, "Determination + Discipline + Hard Work = The Way to Success." I put that formula under the clock because my students have a tendency to look at the clock during class time. As soon as I see a student look at the clock I say, "Are you looking at the clock?" "Nope," is the usual answer. "Did you read that?" I ask. "No, I did not," the student answers. "Read it then," I say. "What does it say? It says 'Determination.' Determination means you refuse to quit. You don't give up, Johnny. It also says, 'Discipline.' Discipline means you are full of instructions from your mom, your dad, and your coach. I'm just the coach. Remember that the coach is only as good as the team, and you are the best. What else does it say?" Johnny says, "Uh, hard work." "Yes," I say to him. "Hard work—it makes the future. You are the future. The only thing I am asking from you is that you believe in yourself. If you believe in yourself, you build confidence. If you believe in yourself, you think positively. If you believe in yourself, Johnny, it's a step to success. You can do it. Anybody can do it."

The other day a fellow teacher told me this story. During his first year of teaching two boys named Johnny were in his class. One was a happy child and an excellent student. The other Johnny spent much of his time goofing off and making a nuisance of himself. The teacher suspected that the second Johnny would be a problem all year.

Toward the end of September the PTA held its first meeting of the year. A mother came up to my friend the teacher and said, "How's my son Johnny getting along?" For some reason my friend assumed she was the good Johnny's mother and said, "I can't tell you how much I enjoy him. I'm so glad he's in my class." The next day the problem Johnny went up to his teacher and said, "My mom told me what you said about me last night. I didn't know any teacher ever wanted me."

That day the problem Johnny did the classwork. The following day he brought in his homework. A few weeks later he became a good friend of his teacher's, and eventually he became one of the best students in the class. I think sometimes we mistake the identity of a person by believing he is just a loser and will always be a loser. We give up on some of our students. I tell my students that they must combine their intelligence with intuition and a great deal of hard work in order to succeed. I tell them not to be afraid to try to succeed and that successful people make many mistakes and then learn from them. Abraham Lincoln lost several elections before he won the Presidency. We must not lose hope in our students, and we need to encourage them not to lose hope in themselves.

Our teenage students need hope and challenge. In life we all face different kinds of problems, and it is difficult to say that any particular solution is going to work. That's why I say to my students, "You can do it. Anybody could do it." One Sunday in church my pastor told a story about Babe Ruth playing a game in Chicago. He said, "Babe Ruth hit two home runs in that game. But the thing that is really exciting is that in that game, Babe Ruth had two strikes. Ruth struck out many times in his life, maybe fifteen hundred times. In this game in Chicago, a pitch came to Babe Ruth. He extended his arm, took the swing, and the ball went flying over the outfield fence. Pandemonium broke loose in the stadium. His teammates carried him across the field. They picked him up and let him down so he could touch the first base, then the second base, third base, and home. The game was stopped for twenty minutes as the crowd responded to Babe Ruth's home run, and it was only the fourth inning. At the end of the game the reporters were questioning Babe Ruth, and one of them asked, 'What would you have done if you had not hit a home run? What would you have done if you had struck out?'

"People present say that Ruth looked stunned by the question, as though the reporter were out of his mind. He looked at the reporter and replied, 'Mr. Reporter, it never entered my mind to do anything else but hit that home run'."

That is the kind of thinking I expect from my students. "Johnny, hit that home run. But don't feel comfortable; don't feel you're doing your best. People are always looking at you, learning from you. You are the best—you can do it. But don't relax and get comfortable." I expect my students to be winners. If a teacher expects students to be losers, they will lose. If you expect more from your students and hold them accountable, they will offer you more. They will amaze you.

I have seen this at Garfield High School where I taught in Los Angeles. Kids who had been involved in gangs and had no interest in education went on to become doctors. Many became positive people within our society. The teachers played an important role in enabling the students to make positive moves, to stand and deliver. I ask my students where the future is. The future is in chemistry, physics, biology, computer science, electronics. The language of the future is mathematics. The students do not on their own see the relationship between what they are learning in the classroom and what they will be doing in life. Teachers need to help them see that relationship.

Students are not aware that mathematics is the building block to a challenging career in our high-tech society. I tell my students that much of Japan's success is due to the fact that its blue-collar workers are able to interpret advanced mathematics, read complex blueprints, and perform sophisticated tasks on the factory floor. These workers do much better than our American workers, and they do so because they have had a simple, strong background in science, with appropriate discipline and responsibility.

The children of the American barrio have enormous obstacles to overcome in order to get an education. Most of the families of the children I taught at Garfield High School in East Los Angeles have incomes below the poverty level. The majority of the parents have not been to college. Frequently, the parents have never been to high school, and they may or may not appreciate the long-term value of education. My students were naturally affected by these barriers, but they did not have to be victims of them. Students can learn to overcome any barriers they face. With the right kind of hope and challenge and *ganas*, they can conquer all.

A student came to me saying she did not understand the work. I said, "You don't understand? Wonderful—I don't understand either, but you're going to help me understand. Can you read the problem?" The student Maria said, "I'm telling you, I don't understand." I said, "That's exactly what I mean. I don't understand either. If we work together, you're going to be able to understand."

Sometimes a student has a negative attitude towards mathematics, especially girls. Maria said, "Kimo, I can't do it. It's too difficult. I try. I put *ganas*. But I can't do it." So, I used one of my tricks. I said to her, "Tomorrow we're going to be working in groups, and you will be the leader." Exasperated, she said, "I told you: I don't understand it!!! How can I be the leader?!!" I told her, "Don't worry about it. I want you to come in in the morning, and I want to tell you what I'm going to do during the day. In doing it with the class, I will make a mistake. I will go over it with you before class, and you will correct me when I make the mistake."

The next day Maria arrived early and we went over the lesson exactly. Later, in class I went to the chalkboard, made a mistake, and acted confused about the lesson. I asked the class if anyone could help me out. Maria volunteered. That is how I develop a student's confidence. At the end of the day Maria came to me and said, "How did I do?" I said, "Wonderful!" She said, "Kimo, can I ask you another question?" "Go ahead." "Are you going to make another mistake?" "I'm going to make many mistakes, believe me." Maria's confidence was stronger, so her *ganas* could flourish. Teachers teach much more than mathematics, chemistry, or physics.

"*Ganas* is all I need" is the motto I taught my students from the barrio. Once one has *ganas*, learning becomes easy. In English *ganas* translates as "desire." It is much more than that. It is the powerful urge to get ahead, willingness to sacrifice and work hard. *Ganas* is a desire that must emerge from within. I teach my students that with *ganas* they will get to college if they want to. The *ganas* will empower their dreams and enable them to overcome any barriers they face in life.

I teach my students the art of keeping cool under pressure. Pressure can be a great teacher, an energizer. I teach my students that with *ganas* they will learn to use that energy to their own advantage. I urge them to find *ganas* in their lives, something they like, something that captures their imaginations, something they can do to help others improve our country.

Some educators hold the racist notion that Hispanic students are not as smart as some other students and that they shy away from courses that require hard work. I have found that to be completely false. When a student of any race, ethnicity, or economic status is expected to work hard, he or she will usually rise to the occasion and become devoted to the task. *Ganas* requires team effort. The teacher must contribute expectations for hard work and success. Our expectations affect whether our students become winners or losers. Negative racist expectations create losers. Most colleges do not train teachers to deal with students from different ethnic groups. The way to deal with one group is different from the way to deal with another, and I'm learning about that in the school where I teach now, Hiram Johnson High School in Sacramento, where the classes have students from various ethnic groups. However, with students from all ethnic groups, parents and teachers need to work together and need to maintain hope. If parents and teachers hold high expectations for young people, the young will rise to meet them.

Ganas can be cultivated. It can be cultivated through team effort. It is not an easy task, but parents, friends, religious leaders, school administrators, and teachers must all become involved. It is not easy, but it is a requirement. Giving our young people high expectations and admiration will inspire them to believe in themselves. Once they believe in themselves, anything is possible. "You are the best, Johnny. You can do it. People are watching you, looking at you, learning from you. You are an inspiration. This is a great country and you can be anything you want to be. You are our best hope for the future."

I believe in God; I believe in my friends; I believe in my students; and I believe in education. We depend on education to prepare an educated work force and to transmit our cultural heritage to new generations. We depend on education to build the character of our youth. School is the site of world dreams and our opportunities as individuals. Each of us remembers a great teacher, a teacher who touched our lives, gave us encouragement, pushed us to do our best. As a teacher I want to exhibit deep love and care for my students, convey my passion for the subject I teach, and constantly improve my teaching through learning from my mistakes. I am proud to be a teacher. I do not make talents; I discover them. They come in different colors, sizes, and weights. You will find them in any of our schools.

Photograph

SANDI SCHAFFER

On the wall behind my desk in Portable A-3, there are photographs of my students. They pose in groups, smiling or lips tight. There is Minh from Vietnam, with fawn eyes, a tilt to his head, a broad grin. Saba from Eritrea, her river-stone skin in sharp contrast to Eva's olive-brown face. Both girls could be models. Saba's eyes glisten. Eva's have sorrow in them. I have placed the pictures there to add some interest for the students, and to help me learn their names.

This is my second year of teaching Sheltered English Science at a large, urban junior high school, and my classes, a multicultural pot-pourri, resonate with the sounds of distant places, foreign lands.

My room is isolated, outside, away from the main building. At about eye level, a row of eight windows opens onto the yard. The view, a beige stucco wall and asphalt, does not inspire, but the breeze that blows in gives a sense of freshness. When the door is open, as I like it to be, I can see one of the three trees protruding up from the concrete in the school yard. Pruned severely every year, it always manages to bloom forth with a canopy of green leaves as if in defiance of the surrounding landscape. Right now it is bare.

Inside the building African-Americans, Latinos, Asians, and a handful of others tumble along the hallways in the five-minute passing time before the first bell. I am known by many more students than my own. Often my hands have grabbed the backs of shirts to stop fights. I say, "Good morning," "Have a nice weekend," and "That's a great outfit!" Admonishments come snapping out, too, respectful but clearly meant, for littering, cussing, and being late to class.

"We're just playing," the students mutter.

"It's not playing to me," I say. "It hurts when you hit someone. Keep your hands off." They come to my portable for Kleenex and bandaids, and for candy from the big red tin. Everett came once.

Tall and lanky with milk chocolate skin, Everett came to ask about the yearbook contest. We talked about the theme. He liked my room and said so.

"Are a lot of kids entering the contest?" he wanted to know. "I don't draw all that well."

"Go ahead and do it," I said. "Here's a piece of poster board. Do you have markers? Here, take these. Bring your drawing to me Monday." He looked at me for a moment, thinking.

"You're very kind," he said. "Thank you."

"See you Monday."

He left the portable, and I could see his head above the lunchtime crowd as he strode purposefully across the yard. "Kind," I thought. "How easy to be kind." He didn't win the contest, but he always said "hello" to me and smiled in his friendly way.

That day in March, as often was the case, the students clustered by the pictures on my board before the first bell rang. There were new ones up, taken when they did a dry ice lab with smoke-filled beakers and inflated balloons.

"Sit down," I said. "You're tardy if you're not in your seat when the bell rings." Like birds at bread, gathered in the park, they scattered into the room taking pictures with them, leaving empty spots on my board. I'd complain, of course, and say it wasn't right to take my pictures. I even put up a sign that said, "Please don't take the pictures." But they felt entitlement, or too enticed by poses of themselves to give them back. So I'd fill the board, and they would empty it slowly.

Pictures for the yearbook I stashed away. One of Eva and her sister was especially nice. Some months had passed since the snapshot on the board. Her eyes had sparkle in them now, and hope.

Today was an assembly schedule. We'd had no notice of the program, but news like that never was passed along. Our new principal and vice-principal were too busy cleaning up, tightening up, and straightening up our school. Detention was in place, parents were called, and suspensions were beginning to decline. We still had fights and cussing in the halls, but change was in the air, and kids were not as cocky to your face.

First period assembly. My class was second sitting, so they worked on planet reports, spreading out posters of Saturn, Uranus, and Mars. The room had the quiet hum of low chatter that can soothe a teacher into thinking all is well. The door was open and the sun shone in—a shaft of light, dust sifting down. Spring again would bring out green on the tree outside. I took pictures of the students drawing, making charts of distances in space and orbits around the sun. It felt good to be a teacher.

"May I have your attention. All students and teachers may now report to the second assembly." My students filed out. I locked the door and followed them. Crowding into the cafetorium was half the student body, jostling, noisy, eager for the show. Sometimes singers came on stage with instruments and rapped or sang the blues. Sometimes students in costumes from other countries danced for us or just walked by with makeup on and flowers in their hair. Today there was a solemn group, women dressed in blue and brown and men in suits. They began to speak.

"We are the Mothers of Murdered Children." They had come, they said, to tell their tales of senseless killings so that more children wouldn't die. There are no windows in the cafetorium. The curtains on our stage are frayed. I listened as one mother spoke about her son, fifteen, she said. He died one night at a party near a place I used to live. He died because some other kid was mad and shot him by mistake. My own son's face was clear to me just then: sixteen; blue eyes. Tears welled up. I stepped outside through a door into the hall and went into the Office to sit down. I've never let my students see me cry.

No sounds were coming from the cafetorium except that mother, weeping now, but talking on and on. "My students," I thought, "will have to stay and listen to stories they should never have to hear." There was no Kleenex anywhere that I could see. The principal, his hair smoothed back and his glasses straight, asked, "Are you okay?"

"I couldn't listen to what she was saying," I said. "It was so sad." And I wiped my tears with my fingers.

"Yes, it is," he said, and he headed back to work. There just wasn't any Kleenex.

For forty-five minutes the parents told their stories, painful ones that left them bitter and in joyless lives. The students listened quietly, applauding softly after each recounting. Some African-American girls sat to one side. One or two were crying. I asked them if they were okay and said I would find them Kleenex. I walked to the back of the cafetorium where screens fold back to open up the space and join it with the

great hall. The front doors are to the left, and they have windows looking out onto the street. I had been so lost in thought, I'd missed something that had happened.

There were policemen in the hall and an ambulance outside.
Now I saw the solemn teachers who were caring for the boy. Some students from the first assembly had been roaming, weren't in class.
They'd caught the boy and kicked him down: too good, "acting white,"
he made them angry.

They talked on and on, the mothers and fathers in their suits, of
senseless murder while behind us in the hall, a boy, Everett, lay trembling, bruised, and cold. He told the names, six names of those maraud-
ing boys who beat him, and they were rounded up and taken to the
principal. Word travels fast in junior high, and more girls were crying,
Everett's friends. When the medics wheeled the gurney out, the children turned around because they could see the hall, and they stared. A
beaten boy behind them; mothers weeping ahead. On all sides. In their
school. In their city. In their lives.

What had begun like any other day at Lakeview was now the saddest one I've had there. In my classes we talked, my students and I. We
wrote "violence" on the board so we could make some sense of it. We
wrote lists, definitions, and solutions. I made them work, and think of it,
and keep their minds still hopeful. Outside there were other fights,
smaller ones, and girls crying like kittens. After a break on the yard, my
students scurried to our room across the yard like rabbits on the run. I
closed the door but kept the windows open. The breeze came in and
cleaned the air a bit. How could we live with all this violence and still
be safe? We thought of ways and wrote them, too. Eva told of how her
father drank and used to beat her, but a counselor made him stop. Now
I knew what change I'd seen in her eyes.

Eva's story gave us hope, and then she cried. I put my arm around
her, and so did Saba with the river-stone skin. Sitting next to her, Minh,
his deer eyes glistening, wanted me to take a picture of the whole class.
So I did. The children together, against violence. I will make an enlarge-
ment.

I learned that Everett had bruises on his brain and a neck injury,
but would be okay. I was glad to see him later, back at school. The boys
who attacked him were suspended. The photograph I took that day is
on the board. No one has taken it.

The Corrosion of Care in the Context of School

ANNA E. RICHERT

My mother, who is in her eighties now, used to be a nurse. When my sister, brother, and I were growing up she would fill our heads with stories about how nurses and doctors and teachers did things to help people and make them feel better. Thankfully, since I did not spend much time in a hospital or the doctor's office as a child, the only place I could check out my mother's contention about the caring nature of these special adults was in school where I encountered lots of teachers over the years. I've found my mother is right about most things; she was right about teachers. They were helpful to me as I was growing up. And though I don't recall feeling particularly bad, I remember them making me feel better too.

Those early lessons of my mother's about teachers and teaching carried me right through my own schooling to my becoming a teacher myself. Now I teach teachers. I think a lot about what teachers need to know and be able to do to care for kids the way I remember my teachers caring for me. The world is a very different place now, however, from how it was when I grew up. And the care that is needed for children in school by school personnel is of a different order as well. The care that teachers are asked to provide children includes not only teaching them to be good citizens, to think, to read, and to do mathematics, but how to speak English, how to survive the violence of their neighborhoods, how to resist drugs, how to eat properly, how to raise children.

At the core of teaching practice that would help kids grow in these ways is care—care for the child and his or her well-being in this uncertain, rapidly changing, tumultuous world. For children to learn, they need to feel and be safe; this includes needing to trust others, and having a sense that others believe in them. Children need care and they also need to learn to care for one another. Ultimately, they need to learn to care for themselves.

Providing care for children has always been an important function of schooling. It has become increasingly important in recent times, however, when the structure of society and its institutions are undergoing rapid change, and the work of raising children appears to be a protected function of no one. Poverty affects increasing numbers of families, especially families who live in urban centers. In Oakland, California, for example, close to 50 percent of the children served by public schools live with families that qualify for aid to dependent children according to the 1991 Oakland Unified School District Report. Resources are as scant here as is an adequate knowledge base for raising children under poverty's associated conditions of violence, uncertainty, and change.

The African saying, "it takes a village to raise a child," reminds us that child rearing is too complex an enterprise to accomplish alone. However, with the exception of the institution of school, recent times have left the American family all but abandoned for child-rearing help by social service institutions. As the family's capability to perform the work of primary care for children has diminished due to economic and social pressures, the school has assumed a larger role for raising kids. In many urban settings, school is the most predictable and safest place in the child's life.

In response to this expanded role, combined with the rapidly growing and increasingly diverse group of school-aged children needing to be raised, school organizations have become more bureaucratic in their structure. The problem with large bureaucratic organizations in regard to care is that they tend to separate people from one another. Beyond that, processes that value efficiency are heralded at the cost of those that are time-consuming and labor-intensive, such as are required for the giving of care. Equally problematic in terms of giving care is the tension created between the school's mandate to operate according to rational and standardized systems that honor diversity and equity on the one hand, and the caregiving needs that are often individual and nonsystematic on the other.

In this chapter I look at schools and consider how their bureaucratic structure works against an ethical ideal of care. I begin the chapter with a story told to me recently by a teacher colleague who was a student of mine before he became a secondary social studies teacher in the city where we both now work. Nate's[1] story is not unlike several I hear every day in my work as a teacher educator. Using this story as a catalyst, I will present what I consider to be the features of schooling that seem to paralyze schools in enacting their mission of care. I will end the chapter by presenting a model of reflective practice that offers teachers and teacher educators a way to begin to put the heart back into schooling in spite of the extraordinarily difficult circumstances that define school life. It is with this vision of reflective practice that I believe teachers can reconnect with the reasons they entered the profession, and the hope of creating an image of care to guide practice in school and the world that surrounds it.

NATE'S STORY

Nate is a first-year teacher currently teaching in an inner city school in a large metropolitan area. Like most of his novice colleagues, Nate expressed considerable doubt and uncertainty at the outset of his first year teaching. "I hope I can deliver the goods to these kids," he wrote in a letter, "but I'm full of doubts and feeling completely overwhelmed right now."[2] Feeling overwhelmed at the beginning of a new career is understandable for any new teacher. What is less understandable is the lack of support Nate experienced as a newcomer to his profession and school. Symptomatic of the lack of support were the extraordinary number of bureaucratic responsibilities assigned to Nate his first week on the job. "Buried under a mountain of bureaucratic paper demands," he ended that week grasping for the vision that had motivated him to leave his prior career at the age of 44 and become a high school history teacher. As he dreamed about his new job, Nate imagined spending the first weeks getting to know both his students and his new colleagues. Instead, he spent it trying to keep track of kids, answering questions (for which he did not have the answers), filling out forms that corresponded to the high numbers of students he encountered each day. He explained in his letter:

> They want six-weeks of lesson plans, classroom management plans, seating charts, a grading policy, five emergency lesson plans, educational objectives, standards of achievement, my curriculum plan for the entire year (in less than a week!) and, of course, all sorts of forms, transcripts and what-not for the district office.

In spite of these demands, Nate was determined to start his first year teaching by establishing relationships with his students. He organized his school day so that he was able to talk with students and begin what he promised himself would become growing connections over time. One such student was Tyrone Washington, a student in Nate's third period class. In their first conversation Nate asked Tyrone what he planned to do after high school. Tyrone explained that he was returning to school after dropping out over a year ago, and that he "wanted to become a child psychologist so he could help kids like himself who had troubles growing up."

Unfortunately, Tyrone's relationship with Nate was short-lived; he did not come to Nate's class after the first two days of the semester. Nate explained in his letter that one frustration of his first weeks at school came from his inability to find the time to investigate why Tyrone was not in class. The demands of accomplishing what the school situation required overshadowed his commitment to create and sustain relationships in his classroom. There was so much for Nate to do—so many students transferring in and out, so many questions to answer, so much need for guidance from kids who have nowhere else to turn, so many homeroom advisees to plan programs for, so many forms to complete—that Nate lost track of his own priorities. In this commotion he did not check with the office or talk with the administration about Tyrone's absence. Nor did they talk with him. Instead, he properly recorded Tyrone's absence on the proper form that he sent to the office at the proper time each day. Nate explained in his letter that as he completed the absentee form for Tyrone, he worried about him and wondered where he was and why he was not in class given how eager he was that first day. Nate contemplated his own naivete; after all, he had been told numerous times that kids in the inner city miss school over half the time on average.

The nature of Nate's concern took a different course when he serendipitously encountered the school's Dean in the hallway the second week of school. Amidst the confusion of the hallway—which Nate described as matched only by the confusion he felt in his heart—Nate was told by the Dean in a "matter of fact way" that Tyrone was the victim of a shooting incident sometime during that first week of school. In this brutal and yet nonmalicious way Nate learned that Tyrone was not attending his class because he was not alive to do so.

MAKING SENSE OF THE UNSENSEMAKABLE

The tragedy of Tyrone's premature death extends far beyond the scope of this chapter. What is not beyond its scope, however, is what we can learn from these painful events about creating a context of care in school settings. What does this story tell us about school as a context of care? What does it suggest for people like Nate and Tyrone who have chosen to spend a good portion of every day there? We learn from this story, for example, of the possible costs of creating schools so large that knowing one another is rendered impossible. We learn also of the dangerous circumstances of children's lives and are forced to consider how those dangers might become part of what happens in school. Similarly, we learn that adequate schooling cannot be accomplished in isolation of community; it is simply too complex a job for any one institution—family, school or church alike—to raise a child alone. And finally, we learn of the importance of creating a caring heart for teachers as well as students. If we expect schools to be contexts of care, we have to concern ourselves with how to care for the caretakers as well as the children in their charge.

Perhaps we might begin by considering these factors in reverse order. In telling Nate's story, I run the risk of unfairly implicating teachers and other school personnel in the corrosion of care in schools. Suggesting that school adults cause this phenomenon is like suggesting that Red Cross workers in war-stricken countries are the cause for the pain and suffering of the people there. Teachers are not the cause of the decline of care in schools. In fact, in most instances teachers are the reason that caring exists at all in these institutions. In Nate's story, for example, I learned later that the Dean who in the "matter-of-fact" tone informed Nate of Tyrone's death was new to the school herself; she was totally overwhelmed with her new work in this troubled school setting. At the time of this writing, Tyrone was one of fourteen students at the school killed during the school year.

The public school mandate to serve all children, including children whose lives are exceedingly difficult outside of school, puts an enormous strain on teachers who have neither the life experience of many of these children, nor the knowledge of how to be helpful. Finding ways to understand the worlds of children has always posed a dilemma for teachers; the process has never been easy. But the world of children today is often so completely unfamiliar to the teachers who teach them, that even locating points of access is extraordinarily difficult, let alone gaining access once the points are determined. Gael, a recent student of mine, described a confusion similar to Nate's as she planned to teach ninth grade English in an inner city classroom. "Nothing in my experience had prepared me for this," she wrote (Gael, Case Paper, 1992). She explained her feelings:

I had never really been among disenfranchised people before. And I had certainly never even conceived of living on a day to day basis with the level of violence that these students came home to. A girl in the homeroom across the hall stabbed her mother to death by plunging a knife into her forty times. When my most rage-full student finally began to write, it was about the pain of being an unwanted child. These students had the wariness and acuity of people living in a war zone. They fought me on trust issues every step of the way. And somehow, in this foreign country, I had to find a way for us to talk about reading and writing together. (Gael, Case Paper, 1992)

Creating a context of care in schools must include caring for teachers like Nate and Gael. Teachers need support in dealing with the life and death issues that regularly make their way into classrooms. They need assistance in making sense of the events of kids' lives and how they might deal with those events in the school day. They need to feel they are not alone in struggling with these difficult issues, and accept that the uncertainty surrounding their experience is endemic to teaching rather than a condition caused by their own inadequacy.[3] The model of reflective practice proposed later in this chapter is one way to provide such support for teachers. Bringing teachers into conversation about their work with themselves and with others honors relationship in teaching and thus suggests a context of care for those charged with giving care in school settings.

At the core of this conceptualization of care for teachers is relationship—finding ways for teachers to relate to one another and to others. Reducing isolation is fundamental to creating a context of care in school. The other issues raised by Nate's story can similarly be understood in terms of relationship. As schools have taken on more responsibility for raising children (including taking *in* more students in the first place), they have become more bureaucratized. Institutions with complex structures typically function to separate people from one another rather than bring them together. While this arrangement and its consequence may be appropriate in an industry where product rather than people is of primary concern (and I am not convinced of the appropriateness in these settings either), it is devastating in school settings where the work is for and about children and their lives in our complex world.

Just as Nate needed more opportunity to connect with his Dean over the circumstances of Tyrone's death (and she with him), he also needed more time to come to know both Tyrone and Tyrone's classmates. Cornel West (1993) in his provocative book on race, discusses the importance of community and connection for derailing the pervasive nihilism that threatens black (and I would argue poor) America. Defining nihilism as "the lived experiences of coping with a life of horrifying meaninglessness, hopelessness, and (most important) lovelessness," West warns of the result:

> a numbing detachment from others and a self-destructive disposition toward the world. Life without meaning, hope, and love, breeds a cold hearted, meanspirited outlook that destroys both the individual and others (pp. 14–15).

It is absolutely essential that we rethink schools in ways that honor the core value of relationship. Teachers' professional relationships with one another, their relationships with children, the children's relationships with one another, relationships with parents, with other community members, are all critical to creating school in the image of care. Schools must be reorganized so that all people in the community served by the school can know and care for one another. Smaller classes, different schedule arrangements that bring people together for longer amounts of time, structures that reinvite and otherwise support community involvement, are all strategies for bringing people back together and thus restore meaning, hope, and love into the lives of people who attend school and who need to be cared for in this presence.

REFLECTIVE TEACHING AND THE CONTEXT OF CARE

Embracing a model of reflective teaching is one way to advance the cause of care in schools. Unlike more traditional models of teaching in which the teacher is primarily a holder and dispenser of knowledge, reflective teachers are assumed, rather, to be creators and definers of knowledge. Additionally, reflective teaching assumes that central to good teaching is a rigorously thoughtful examination of the purposes and consequences of what teachers do. The actual reflective process occurs frequently in teaching and refers to those times when action is stopped, even temporarily, and the teacher (either alone or with others) attempts to make sense of what has occurred, what is occurring, what will occur. The knowledge that results from this inquiry guides further practice. The model values experience as an important source of knowledge about teaching and the teacher as the holder of that experience, the valued knower.

Given its reliance on experience as a cornerstone, reflective teaching offers a context of hope for reinstituting care as the primary tenet of school practice. There are several reasons why I believe this is so. The first concerns the complexity of school settings as discussed earlier in this chapter. Schools and their surrounding communities are extraordinarily complex entities partially due to the rapidly changing economic and social conditions that surround them. No one better than those directly involved in the world of schools can imagine or even hope to come to know the impact of change on school life in terms of creating schools as caring, learning environments for children.

Reflective teaching requires, by definition, an ongoing examination of what *is* in school settings, as compared with what might be or ought to be. Teachers, who have chosen to be on the front line, are entrusted with the responsibility of examining the real and changing circumstances of school life—every moment, every day, every year—as they work to create schools where everyone can learn. Without care, learning cannot occur. Without this first-hand, rigorous examination of the actual conditions of school, the possibility of creating that caring context is lost.

The process of honest "naming," which is that of reflective teaching, is the second reason I believe this teaching model offers hope for generating care in school settings. Reflective teaching assumes that teachers are the "experts" about teaching practice. Their expertise comes from a reflective cycle of naming, analyzing, and acting in an intelligent and morally responsible way. As teachers engage in this reflective process, they work to define the circumstances of their school settings, and then plan and act from that place of knowing. The reflective process allows them to be authentically responsive to the communities they serve. The alternative model of teaching in which expertise is seen as outside school practice (and usually delivered from the university research community or local or state governmental organizations), is much less likely to touch the real needs of the people in school. Without an authentic connection, the capacity for care is compromised.

Reflective teaching requires that teachers embrace the inherent uncertainty of schooling, and deal honestly with the sometimes troubling condition of social life and its impact on school experience. Through self-determined examination and action, teachers claim ownership of their work, and, therefore, the ability to create school worlds as they believe these worlds should be. The task requires that reflective teachers know the community of the school and incorporate into their reflective conversation and contemplation the voices of those directly on the other side of the school wall. Reflective teaching does not happen in isolation. In fact, reflection requires that teachers work with others to examine school life and practice. Reflective knowledge is local knowledge because it is generated from a reflective examination of experience; local, rather than generalized or abstracted knowledge, offers the opportunity of breaking down barriers between school and community. This is a third reason I believe reflective teaching offers hope for creating schools in a new image.

The fact that reflection does not happen in isolation presents an additional factor connecting reflective teaching as care in schools. As a process, reflection is ubiquitous in good teaching; successful teachers constantly inquire about what they do in the classroom, and why. While some of this thinking necessarily happens alone, a great potential for it happening in the company of others is part of the model of reflective teaching I am proposing here. Recently I have had the experience of examining a variety of models of reflective teaching for both novice and experienced teachers (see Richert 1992a, 1992b; 1991). The factor about this approach to teaching that captured the spirit and interest of these teachers with whom I had this contact was the sense of professional identity, commitment, and community the process engendered.

Earlier in this chapter I spoke of the need for caring for the caretakers if we want to create a community of care in school settings. Creating a culture of inquiry that supports reflective process will create an environment of care for teachers. Dewey reminded us years ago that teaching is an intellectual rather than a technical task. A model of reflective practice challenges teachers to honestly engage their full intellectual and emotional selves as they work to make sense of their experiences in school settings. The process allows them to act with intent and to think and act with intent with others. As teachers work together to confront the inordinately complex and extraordinarily difficult circumstances of school life, they seize the power of coming to

know and the hope of coming to act in caring ways. Our hope for rein-
venting schools that care for children is in creating schools that care
for teachers by supporting them in doing the work they are called
upon, prepared for, and capable of doing. In this way we can begin to
restore care as the essential quality of school life for the twenty-first
century.

REFERENCES

Janofsky, Gael, A Case of Less Being More. Unpublished case manuscript.
    Mills College, 1992.
McDonald, Joseph P., *Teaching: Making Sense of an Uncertain Craft* (New York:
    Teachers College Press, 1992).
Richert, A. E., "Voice and Power in Teaching and Learning to Teach," in *Reflec-
    tive Teacher Education: Cases and Critiques*, Valli, L., ed. (London: Falmer
    Press, 1992).
Richert, A. E., "Enhancing the Reflection of Beginning Teachers by Structur-
    ing Opportunities for Considering Broader Content," in *Teachers and
    Teaching: From Classroom to Reflection*, Munby, H. and Russell, T., eds.
    (London: Falmer Press, 1992).
Richert, A. E., "Using Cases for Reflection and Enhanced Understanding," in
    Staff Development: New Demands, New Realities, New Perspectives, 2nd Edi-
    tion, Lieberman, A., and Miller, L., eds. (New York: Teachers College
    Press, 1991).
West, Cornel, *Race Matters* (Boston: Beacon Press, 1993).

NOTES

1. The name Nate is a pseudonym as are the names of other former students I refer to in this chapter. The purpose of this is to provide them anonym-
ity. The stories I include in the chapter, however, have not been altered.

2. The quotes in this example are from a letter Nate wrote in September, 1992, several weeks into his new teaching position.

3. For a powerful discussion of the uncertainties of teaching and the
role of uncertainty in undermining a teacher's confidence and self-esteem, see
Joseph McDonald's *Teaching: Making Sense of an Uncertain Craft* (1992) New
York: Teachers College Press.

Death by Choice

Theresa Stephany

In his youth Luke had been a professional dancer. He had danced in floorshows in Reno and Las Vegas and in a Miss America Pageant hosted by Bert Parks himself! By the time we met, Luke's brain tumor had rendered him completely immobile from the neck down. Quadraplegia is a nightmare for any patient, but it seemed a particularly cruel fate for a man who had made his living from movement.

I had heard about Luke and his wife Jean from my patient who lived next door to them. I knew that I would be Luke's home care hospice nurse whenever he was ready for hospice. I also knew that Jean was an R.N., so I thought there was no need to push the referral. I felt lucky to have a patient whose primary caregiver was a nurse. I knew that my own job would be much easier with a nurse around twenty-four hours a day. I was, indeed, fortunate to have Jean at Luke's side. Later, I wished I had known how sick Luke was and what a heavy load she had been carrying for so long.

When I met Jean and Luke, I was amazed at the excellent care Jean had been providing. Insulin-dependent all his life, Luke had no problems that revealed his diabetic condition. He had no skin breakdown, no contractures, no indwelling catheters, not even a hospital bed or a Hoyer lift. He slept and eventually died in his own bed next to the wife who loved him passionately and took superb care of him. I was both in awe of and completely horrified by their sad situation.

Luke hated every moment of his existence. Unlike his neighbor who thanked God for each additional day of life, Luke cursed Him. He *begged* his wife and daughter to kill him and despaired because he could no longer pick up his rifle and shoot himself. "If you loved me," he would say to Jean, "you wouldn't let me suffer like this." He'd say it over and over again. Luke asked everyone who came to their house to end his misery by killing him. Friends and neighbors stopped visiting.

119

Even their daughter stayed away leaving Jean to shoulder the caregiving burden alone.

My first visit to Jean and Luke was a lengthy one and by the time I left them I was overwhelmed with grief. Human hearts were not meant to carry that much pain!

The next day I reluctantly dragged myself back to their front door. I knew things were going to be hard, but I had no idea just how hard they would get. Jean was sobbing in a crumpled heap on the den couch when I arrived. She told me that Luke had been pleading with her to kill him every moment since I'd left their home the day before. Because she was a nurse, Jean knew how it could be done. "It's precisely *because* I'm a nurse that I can't deliberately kill him," she wept. "I know he's miserable and I love him dearly, but killing is against everything I've ever believed in . . . and I'm not God!"

Jean and I knew that because Luke was a hospice patient there would be no autopsy after his death. Two types of insulin and plenty of syringes were in the refrigerator. Jean could easily induce a fatal diabetic coma and without an autopsy no one would know how Luke had died. Luke also had two pints of liquid morphine sulphate 40mg/cc at his bedside. Unaccustomed as he was to the drug, if he drank the bottles he might have a respiratory arrest and die. However, Luke was completely paralyzed and couldn't end his life. And Jean would not intentionally overdose him.

Luke was in despair, and Jean seemed headed for a nervous breakdown. It was a crisis. I wondered if I was overstepping my bounds, but I decided to take a risk and speak to Jean, not as nurse to nurse, but as hospice nurse to distraught spouse. "Jean," I said, "I understand that you cannot do anything that would hasten his death, but may I have your permission to speak frankly with Luke about another option?" Without hesitation she nodded her consent, and we went to find Luke.

At their kitchen table that day I had one of the most honest and gut-wrenching discussions I have had in my seventeen years as a nurse. Because I have been a hospice nurse for a long time I thought I was no stranger to pain. Luke and Jean taught me otherwise. Slowly and deliberately I explained to Luke that he was tearing his wife apart by constantly asking her to kill him. "She loves you more than I can say, but she simply cannot help you end your life. You must stop asking her. It is destroying her. I know you love her back, so let's talk about the options that you do have and really lay it all out on the table. Okay?"

Luke was eager to proceed, so I spoke of the insulin and the morphine—excellent ways to kill oneself but not ones available to him because he couldn't administer the drugs to himself. We spoke of his rifle. He couldn't pull the trigger. Jean was choking on her tears as I listed the unavailable options they had already considered.

I knew that at least one more option did exist. Several months earlier Luke's brain tumor had caused him to have a grand mal seizure. Since that time he had been taking Dilantin orally three times a day. If he elected to stop taking his medications, there was a good chance that the seizures would begin again. Left untreated, seizuring could cause death. "Luke, do you understand what I just said?" I asked. A single tear ran down his cheek as he nodded. "Is this what you want to do?" I asked. He nodded again. Crying too hard to speak, Jean nodded her agreement.

It was over. I had spoken the unspeakable. Wondering if I had done the right thing, I left, promising to visit every day as moral support. Driving to the next patient's home, I thought more about what I had said. I wondered if I was crazy, if I had broken any law, if I would ever practice as a nurse again. Those few minutes were intensely painful and panic-filled for me, but, believing that the die was cast, I settled in for the long haul with this couple.

The next morning I arrived at my desk early to catch up on paperwork. I was shocked to get a call from Jean who told me that Luke had just died. In my worst nightmares I could not imagine the night they had just spent. When I arrived at their house, Luke was still warm, still in his own bed, still with his head and upper body cradled in Jean's arms. As she stroked his head, she told me the story.

After I left their home, Luke stopped taking all medications and went to bed. He had made up his mind and was ready. He asked Jean to come to bed with him and made her promise not to call for help, even for help from the Hospice Unit. They spent the night as they always did, with Jean hugging his motionless body. About three o'clock Luke woke and began having small seizures. The seizures became more frequent and more intense. During the seizures Jean enveloped Luke in the circle of her arms. Between seizures when he could hear her, Jean told him she would not move, would not get up. When he was able to speak, he begged her to "Let me get on with this" and not call for help.

Jean did as Luke asked. They spent nearly three hours together facing one seizure after another. As she had promised, Jean held Luke, did not get up, and did not call for help. Jean helped set his tortured body free.

There was no hurry to call the mortuary. For several hours as I sat there, Jean held Luke and stroked his face while I sat on the edge of the bed and wept. Gone were the feelings of uncertainty I had had about whether or not I should have told Luke about his options. I was impaled by the grief of Jean's loss. Also, I knew that my place was in home care hospice, and that I would not be leaving that work. Only a fool would give up a position that allows her to work beside the most courageous and skilled R.N. one could ever hope to meet—my colleague, Luke's wife Jean.

Beyond the Ethics of Rightness: The Role of Compassion in Moral Responsibility

DAVID C. THOMASMA

Since the beginning of modern clinical medical ethics, it has been no secret that the reasoning patterns of clinical judgment in medical care parallel those of ethical judgment.[1,2,3] This realization is important for many reasons. For example, ethics education programs in medical schools have acquired a "clinical" focus of relevance and reality by stressing the similarity between medical and ethical decision making. Articles and books on the philosophy of medicine have sometimes underscored the relation of the ethics of medicine to clinical judgment.[4] More pointedly for our purpose, the nexus between clinical medicine and clinical ethics can help reveal structures of good decision making in medicine that are not simple products of contractual models of the doctor-patient relationship. More is going on in that relationship than initially meets the eye.

I will focus on how the good emerges from medical and clinical judgment, and how the interaction of persons in context leads to that emergence. Put another way, the medical encounter in its context interprets the good through emergent values of doctors, other health providers, and patients. The case often drives our thought, and compassion itself drives the case.

INTRODUCTION

One of the most notable phenomena of recent times is the increasing dissatisfaction of a large portion of human beings worldwide with a materialistic and deterministic worldview. Ironically this dissatisfaction occurs at the very moment in human history that science and technology have been able to advance the cause of human aims and values. People are experiencing increased health and life-spans, decreasing concerns about joblessness, and so on. In many countries persons are provided equal and free access to health care, child care centers for working parents, retirement benefits for workers, and at least some degree of social and family comfort.

The benefits of a materialist culture ring hollow to many persons, who long for a kind of spiritual, cultural, and political freedom. At the heart of this urging is a recognition that the materialist and rationalist worldview does not adequate supply the answers to human reality.[5] Further, the quest is based on a yearning to search and grow oneself. If any reaction occurs cross-culturally today it is that against a sort of smugness, of authority, of those who seem to think that there is some final answer, and that reality can be explained, if they condescend to do so, in some neat, tidy, rationalistic, and complete package.

These urgings not only touch human beings politically; they are also part of the intellectual and personal search for meaning that is found in medicine and other human enterprises. Rather than the broader reaction to the rationalism of the Enlightenment documented elsewhere by such thinkers as MacIntyre,[6] the focus of this paper will be on biomedical decision making.

I will construct an argument that not only rationality, but also emotional compassion, is an important feature of bioethical decision making. Indeed I argue that our compassion can lead us to truths beyond reason and its analysis. In order to do so, I will first examine the powerful divinity-role played by modern medicine in its quest to overcome the exigencies of life and death. Counterbalancing this role is the standard account of rationalistic bioethics that deliberately removes particularity from the decision-making matrix. The purpose of this approach is to find some common ground among persons of varying belief-systems, in order to control biomedical technology's impact on personal autonomy, thus minimizing as far as possible the diversity of individuals and societies. Following a brief examination of this account, I will then discuss the general features of compassionate involvement with the sick and the dying. The concluding section will examine compassionate contextualism, as I call this approach.

PLAYING GOD

Physicians have always used specialized knowledge for the interests of patients. Controlling this knowledge has given the profession and the individual physician great authority in society, in daily affairs, and within the doctor-patient relationship. Modern medical technology empowers individuals beyond their normal capacities. Because technology is, by definition, an extension of human work, it tempts us to exceed the bounds of temperance. This leads to a kind of paternalism in which an individual comes to believe that he or she knows best what is good for another person by employing the powers technology now invests in that individual.

Medical technology adds to this traditional paternalism an even greater temptation, the temptation to "play God." Its opposite, a pusillanimous abandonment of patients without sufficient intervention is found less often, but might appear when inappropriate judgments about either patient values or the patient's quality of life are made.

At the outset it must be admitted that human beings have an incredible thirst for power. Surely this is one reason that humanity is perpetually dissatisfied with the *status quo* and therefore, with the restless attempts at change for the better that characterize our progress through history. General Electric Corporation used to have an advertisement that proclaimed: "Progress is our most important product." Progress in what, one might ask? The answer cannot be just technological improvement. To lead a good life it must include mastery of life's vicissitudes. There is nothing intrinsically wrong with our efforts to improve our lives. On the contrary it is part of the mission of all human beings to use their facilities and propensities to bring about the good in their lives and in society.

Sometimes, however, the lure of "mastery" of the environment, the circumstances of one's life, the future of civilization overwhelms us. It results not in improvements or empowerments for the better, but rather increased dependency, fear, and an "anxiety of possibilities." One example that foreshadows all others in this century is atomic power and its destructive potential. Indeed, for many this represents the modern example of the story of human pride and folly told by the Tower of Babel story in the Old Testament. To build the tower, the human community destroyed itself.

Another example of technology gone amok, and more to our focus on the crisis of care, is that of life-prolonging technology. In this regard, Jonsen wonders just what exactly life support supports: "We talk about the maintenance of life; we don't often talk about the maintenance of personhood. It interests me little," he says, "indeed, not at all, to be alive as an organism. In such a state I have no interests. It is enormously interesting for me to be a person . . . it is the perpetuation of my personhood that interests me; indeed, it is probably my major and perhaps my sole real interest."[7]

Many technologies developed for specific groups of patients are now used for other patient populations where their effect has yet to be evaluated. Because the equipment makes the provider feel better, it is used. When technologies become more accessible, e.g., dialysis, cardiopulmonary resuscitation, there is less of an imperative to justify their use. When ICU beds are plentiful, dying patients are tucked into them.

The effect of overuse of technology without evaluation of its efficacy and, frequently, without patient consent, or even over patient objections, is to increase patient and family suffering. It may prolong the suffering of dying, and it provides social suffering by wasting resources that might benefit those with potentially reversible diseases. The ICU is a prime illustration of both the effective use and the misuse of technology in our society. The cost of an ICU bed is approximately $2,000-3,000 a day.[8] Other hospital beds cost about one-half that amount. Seventy to eighty percent of patients leave the ICU alive. Many of these are postoperative patients. But of those who are critically ill with chronic disease or major medical or surgical problems, the mortality rate is 40-60%. A case in point comes from treatment of AIDS. According to NIH statistics, the mortality rate in ICUs for ventilated AIDS patients is at least 85%. Those with first incidence of pneumonia often benefit from the ICU. Indeed, the ICU is a major benefit to patients for whom it was designed. But the weak or chronically ill will almost certainly die tethered to their machines in that environment for which it was not designed.[9]

In fact, the problem of euthanasia as well as the incredibly difficult questions about human reproduction, and all the others in between the origin of life and the final moment of death, involve the question of dominion over life. Because of our technology, the temptation to take control over life itself is almost overwhelming. In health care, "more" options do not necessarily translate into "better" health care. Thus, mapping the genome will not only increase our store of knowledge about the complexity of the human genetic structure, but will also lead to genetic therapies and, not too far in the future, to interventions to improve this structure before conception itself.

On the other hand, inappropriate withdrawal and withholding of care is also a kind of "playing at God" since it involves one individual, entrusted with the care of another, making judgments about the value of that person's life. It is important to distinguish here between objective evaluation of interventions and outcomes on the well-being of the patient, and subjective quality of life judgments in which the physician judges that the life the patient is now living is not worthwhile.

For the U.S. today the danger exists in the economic sphere.[10] Will it be easier to use a simple method of dispatching those persons whose care costs too much, or who are now considered to be a burden on society, like the aged and the poor, than to address their suffering, which sometimes is overwhelming even for the most dedicated caregivers? As Joseph Cardinal Bernardin noted in an address on euthanasia at the University of Chicago Hospital, "We cannot accept a policy that would open the door to euthanasia by creating categories of patients whose lives can be considered of no value merely because they are not conscious."[11] While morally valid surrogates who express the intent of the incompetent patient about the care in question may make such decisions, the issue does focus on the importance of maintaining compassionate respect for human life in our society. Cardinal Bernardin goes on to pose this question: "What would we be suggesting to one another and to our society, if, seemingly with the best of motives, we were to say that those who are sick, infirm, or unconscious may be killed? How could we allege that such actions would not affect us individually and collectively"?[12] Such actions are a form of "privatizing life," denying its social and communal dimensions as both a private and public good.

Therefore the concerns of disvaluing human life through technical responses to human suffering should not be dismissed as hopelessly conservative and neurotic. The overbearing experience of the twentieth century is one in which persons have been put at the mercy of technology. Caution about this reversal of the creative process, wherein persons are now subject to their own creations, is not only justified, but important in making bioethical decisions.

THE STANDARD ACCOUNT OF SECULAR BIOETHICS

Given the plurality of points of view in bioethics, as in all human affairs, and the constant interplay of viewpoints in public policy, proposals have been made recently that suggest secular humanism ought to be the proper starting point for bioethics consensus. Leaving aside an examination of the role of religious commitment in public policy, which I have done elsewhere with Edmund D. Pellegrino,[13] I will now explore the thesis that enlightened rationality provides the best possible basis for consensus bioethical decision making.

The emphasis upon personal autonomy in medical ethics is coming under greater scrutiny today. Concerns about libertarian assumptions implied by this emphasis have led many thinkers to counter autonomy with the need for beneficence as well.[14,15] The implications of conflicts about medical ethics and ethical theory include the increased role of the health provider's values in caring for the dying patient, greater attention to the relation between physician and patient rather than exclusive focus on the needs and wants of the individual patient alone, and questions about the kind of society we ought to be.

Perhaps the most articulate spokesperson for the libertarian point of view is H. Tristram Engelhardt, Jr. In his *Bioethics and Secular Humanism*, he argues that secular humanism itself has no moral content. But as a contentless position it reigns supreme for moral argumentation among moral strangers, that is, individuals whose fundamental values are either unknown to one another, or actually, whose moral values can be considered to be estranged from one another. In effect, Engelhardt bases his argument on a fundamental rationality all human beings share that can enlighten them in their pursuit of consensual agreements in bioethics.[16]

First it must be acknowledged that the strengths of this position are many. It provides for a rationality and abstract oversight that can relieve one of the particularities of time and place, of commitments and even prejudices, that are part of the everyday moral fiber of individuals, institutions, societies, and governments. Such a "contentless" approach as proposed by Engelhardt, in the end, considers fundamental moral commitments commonly found, for example, among people with a religious faith, as valid only insofar as they can be subject to human rationality. It would be hard not to be sympathetic to any view that espouses enlightened human understanding. Yet the history of thought provides plenty of examples of how rationalistic humanism seems to neglect the emotional side of human experience and the lessons that can be learned from that experience.

That being said, a secular bioethics contains within it seeds of destruction for fundamental commitments. They are, as it were, vacuumed out of the public discussion if and when (as they will almost always be) they are not subject to universalizability, abstraction, and general consensus. In effect, the secular humanism approach that leads to consensus and procedural bioethics tends to destroy moral particularity.[17] Ironically, in its attempt to reach the most public and most common consensus, using secular humanism must become both the most abstract and formal of all bioethics, and the least sensitive to individuality, commitments, contexts, and human relations.[18]

Insofar as some of these particularities, if they can be so called, lead to prejudice and unexamined assumptions, the secular humanism approach advanced by Engelhardt is helpful. It is helpful because it removes such impediments to reason from the public debate. Indeed, Engelhardt is quick to acknowledge that secular humanism need not be inimical to a religious perspective. But this is due less to tolerance of differences and fundamental commitments than to the role of rationality in examining such commitments for what can be publically extracted from them for common consumption.

Another source of caution lies in adopting too readily the rather sunny view of the Enlightenment that hovers in the background of this approach. No less a figure that Benjamin Franklin, early an avowed Deist, became more cautious about this optimistic view of the world and of human affairs when he noticed in himself attributes that shocked him for their negative human characteristics. He had concluded that because of the attributes of God, His infinite wisdom and so forth, nothing could be wrong with the world, and therefore "that Vice & Virtue were empty Distinctions, no such Things existing." But his own conduct toward others made him pause: "I began to suspect that this Doctrine [Deism] tho' it might be true, was not very useful . . . [It] appeared not so clever a Performance as I once thought it."[19]

Any doctrine of human rationality must be met with reservation: our own ineptitude at honoring others, downright evil deeds, and the general violent nature of human society today in every sphere, in which individuals are treated as objects for the pleasure and good of others, indict an unexamined view of human rationality itself. More important for my thesis is the fact that a rationalistic approach to bioethical decision making ignores the embodiment of human beings and their potentialities of nature and virtue to identify with a vulnerable, sick, or dying individual through compassion.

In the end, secular humanism is a faith commitment in it own right. It believes in the ability of human beings to reason out their differences by examining their fundamental commitments dispassionately. Yet such fundamental commitments dilate all the passions toward the end toward which the commitment urges. It is not only the ultimate example of particularity, it also is an ultimate example of passionate thinking, not dispassionate. As Luther said, with a great deal of passion: "Hier stehe ich. I kann nicht anders." "Here I stand. I cannot do otherwise." This is not an ironic position for public consensus or clinical decision making. No amount of dispassionate analysis would bring its confrontational quality to heel.

Some thinkers are concerned with profound arguments about traditional commitments to the value of human life as contrasted to respect for autonomy alone.[20] Thus Leon Kass presents a thoughtful articulation of what is owed a dying patient by the physician. He argues that humanity is owed humanity, not just "humaneness" (i.e., being merciful by killing the patient). Kass argues that the very reason we are compelled to put animals out of their misery is that they are *not* human and thus demand from us some measure of humaneness. By contrast human beings demand from us our humanity itself. This thesis, in turn, rests on the relationship "between the healer and the ill" as constituted, essentially, "even if only tacitly, around the desire of both to promote the wholeness of the one who is ailing."[21]

The temptation to employ technology rather than one's personhood in the process of healing I call "the technological fix." The technological fix is not only easier to conceptualize and implement than the more difficult processes of human engagement, but is also "suggested" by technology itself. The training and skills of modern health professionals are overwhelmingly nurtured within a bath of technological fixes. By instinct and proclivity, all persons in a modern civilization are tempted by technical rather than personal solutions to problems.

THE NATURE OF COMPASSION

Today our attitudes to sickness are vastly different from those in earlier times. Sickness has become a scandal, a contradiction to our frenetic pursuit of the cult of health, youth, and pleasure. We expect medical miracles to exorcise illness. But the sick person is sometimes a brutal reminder of the finitude and frailty we want so much to deny. Rather than being our brothers and sisters, the sick have become alien to us—inhabitants of a world that is no longer ours. In our world, thus, the sick are relegated to hospitals, nursing homes and hospices, away from our immediate presence, so that their plight cannot threaten, or at least minimally threatens, our own sense of power provided by modern technology. Their care is assigned to strangers and professionals. They suffer and die surrounded by the apparatus of technology, often unable to communicate their needs. Their friends and families live at a distance. It is hard even for the most loving individuals to be present for their family members who are sick at the moments of their greatest need.

Traditionally, the community underlined compassionate care of individuals by providing the structures needed for individuals who were sick to be surrounded by those who both loved them the most and also knew their values. Decisions about health care, then, were made within a context of compassion and respect for the values of the patient. The care of such individuals was impervious to marketplace economics. It was an act of mercy, not a commodity to be traded or delivered. Now we worry instead about the resources the sick divert from our other projects. We talk of rationing the care we give, especially to the most vulnerable among us—the poor, the elderly, the chronically handicapped, the infants, the mentally ill, and the retarded. We shrink from the sacrifice—of our time, emotions, energies, and money—that the care of the sick so much requires. So urgent has the economics of health care become that some traditional caregivers, like religious hospitals, even contemplate withdrawing from this vital service.

But none of the changes in society or the technology of medical care can alter the call the sick themselves press upon us so insistently. They call us to see them as fellow creatures in need.[22] This we can do only if we become agents of mercy and compassion. In the effort to be compassionate, we must "permeate and improve the whole society."[23] What is the meaning of this compassion within the context of biomedical decisions?

Compassion is more than pity or sympathy. It transcends social work, philanthropy, and government programs. It is the capacity to feel, and suffer with, the sick person—to experience something of the predicament of illness, its fears, anxieties, temptations, its assault on the whole person, the loss of freedom and dignity, the utter vulnerability, and the alienation every illness produces or portends. True compassion is more than feeling. It flows over in a willingness to help, to make some sacrifice, to go out of one's way. "No one can help anyone without entering with his whole person into the painful situation; without taking the risk of becoming hurt, wounded, or even destroyed in the process."[24]

Compassion entails a comprehension of the suffering experienced by another. When we have suffered ourselves we are sometimes better able to understand it in others. As Unamuno says, "Suffering is the substance of life and the root of personality, for only suffering makes us persons."[25] Compassion for the suffering of others thus enriches our own understanding of what we too must some day pass through. It teaches us that "merciful love is never a unilateral act."[26] Compassion helps us, therefore, to realize that our sick brothers and sisters are not alien to us. They are still very much part of the human family. They are vital to our own spiritual growth. The healthy need the sick to "humanize" them as much as the sick need us to humanize their sickness.

For health professionals and the family or surrogates, compassion is the quality that separates them from objectivity and rationality alone. It enables them to recognize that, effective as our science and technology can be, they do not remove suffering. The sick cannot escape the confrontation with mortality that even a minor illness may entail. Human illness is always illness of the whole person—body, mind, and spirit. Hence, the illness and/or dying process is more than some aberration in an organ system. The illness transcends the biological. It encompasses the whole person and his or her value system. Illness fractures our image of ourselves, upsets the balance we have struck between our aspirations and our limitations. Illness is nothing less than a deconstruction of the self.

Compassion enables the decision makers to assist in healing, if by healing we can mean the reconstruction of the person. Involved here is an effort to put back together a ruptured self that has separated into an ego and a body that has betrayed that individual.[27] We must heal the attack on the spirit as well as the attack on the body. The particularities of culture, ethnicity, language are what makes illness a unique experience for each of us. True healing can only take place when all of these particulars are taken into account.[28] The decisions to be made, then, entail a rich awareness of particulars and values. These decisions, although guided by general, abstract principles, involve the emotions and values of all the parties involved in the process of caring for the sick person.

Compassionate care also means that the patient who cannot be cured by medical sciences—the chronically ill, the mentally retarded, the psychotic—may still be "healed." Even the dying patient can be healed if we help him or her to express the meaning of a life in the final days of that life by respecting, insofar as possible, the values and commitments of that life. Compassion influences the way decision makers would incorporate in decisions the three major principles that dominate medical ethics today—beneficence, justice, and autonomy. It makes all of medical ethics subservient to one ordering principle—acting out of the very particularities of the individual situation.

Thus beneficence must go well beyond the minimalistic interpretation of avoiding harm. It entails helping others even when that involves inconvenience, sacrifice, and risk to our self-interest.[29] This is of urgent importance today when altruism and self-interest so often conflict. We see that conflict in many guises—in physicians refusing to treat AIDS patients for fear of infection or withholding obstetrical and neurosurgical care for fear of malpractice, or acting as medical entrepreneurs, gatekeepers, or striking for higher pay. All of these practices deny the primary obligation of advocacy of the patient's interest, which is at the heart of any compassion-based medical ethic.

Effacement of self-interest is crucial for such decisions by removing worries about damage to career and to institution.[30] With the advent of the Patient Self-Determination Act, many institutions panicked about supplying information to patients about decision making because they saw this as an attack on the doctors' ability to act in the best interests of patients. Yet patients' decisions about their care is one of the best ways to protect their own best interests.

The principle of justice is likewise transformed. It is no longer that strict accounting of what is owed that separates compassion from justice. Mercy is the very essence of it. "True mercy is, so to speak, the most profound source of justice."[31] Compassionate justice is charitable justice with its roots in love for all persons and its fulfillment in a reconstruction of an ideal community in which all persons are treated according to their needs. On this view all humans have just claims on those things society can provide that ensure the dignity of the person and the value of each human life.

Finally, compassion comprehends and respects the moral claim of autonomy. It recognizes the dignity of the sick as full participants in their own healing. We violate the humanity of the sick when, even in the name of benevolence, we ignore their decisions and their spiritual or personal values. This is the very antithesis of the humanization of illness compassion seeks. But this respect for the dignity of choice is not unilateral. The sick person must see the physician and nurse as a brother or sister as well. The patient cannot ask them to violate their moral beliefs. Patient and physician are partners in the act of healing.

COMPASSIONATE CONTEXTUALISM

A responsible use of technological intervention with and for the sake of an individual patient requires not only rational analysis, but also a particular sensitivity to the particularities of the case and the emotional content of value commitments of the parties involved. The responsible use of power is a clinical ethics judgment in every case about the best balance of interventions and outcomes.

The most dramatic examples of taking such responsibility for the particularities of a case are culled from the problems of withholding and withdrawing care from the dying. But compassion is also required to assess properly the interventions to be given to the weak and debilitated elderly, to the demented, to individuals who wish to exercise their autonomy in ways that are easily judged to be self-destructive, and to children, to mention just a few of the challenges presented by modern medicine to both physicians and patients alike.

Casuistry

I am very sympathetic to casuistry as the basic model for how the good decision emerges in medicine. But more work must be done on the assumptions of casuistry. This becomes apparent when we begin to delve into the ways in which medical judgment interprets experience by "mining" the good. There is no time to explore all the ramifications of this kind of question. We can only target two major problems with casuistry.

The most difficult part of casuistry is that it presupposes a unified theory of human nature by which one case can be logically compared to another. This unified theory of human nature was provided by the Natural Law Theory. But this theory, as it was employed in the past, is now as discredited as is traditional casuistry. Toulmin and Jonsen in their book argue that casuistry arose as a method at just that time in Western civilization when the metaphysical superstructure of Christianity began to collapse under the rise of the modern state, nationalism, and the age of reason.[32] They therefore make the case that casuistry is eminently suitable for modern times, times of pluralism, times without a moral consensus.[33] Yet it is difficult to ignore the need for some mode of comparison by which one case is at the very least analogous to the other. Otherwise we are lost in the same dilemma posed by Wittgenstein for which the language games were a solution. Meaning is not wholly and completely individual. It arises in a context beyond or encompassing the individual case. The very basis for analogous cases is some perduring "something" that crosses the boundaries of each case, each ethics-game as it were (to continue the Wittgenstein analogy).

There is a second, and related, problem. When casuistry began to be discredited, it was done so by those who held that ethical theory was very important. The method of ethical analysis changed from case-orientation to deducing practical conclusions from principles. Reinstituting casuistry as the model for both ethical and medical decisions neglects the importance of ethical theory, and analogously, of the relationship of individuals within the case and their values to the emergence of the good.

Contextualism

Just as Kant was awakened from his dogmatic slumbers by reading Hume, and by taking seriously the challenge to science that Hume's skepticism hurled, so too the deductive model of ethical reasoning has been hurled a challenge by casuistry. It is closer to clinical judgment, it describes realistically (rather than ideally) how good decisions come about, and it is practical. Yet it neglects the importance of theory, and of the nexus of values that ethical theory seeks to protect.

Is there a middle ground between deducing the good decision from abstract and theoretical principles that ignore clinical realities, and educing the former entirely from the latter? Is there a middle ground between deduction and induction of the good?

A middle course between a generalist application of ethical theory and specialized case-by-case analysis is possible with a contextual grid for medical ethics.[34] It is only one example of work on contexts to which medical ethics must address itself. Neither axioms nor standard moral rules are sufficient (although they are necessary of course) to determine the validity of moral theory and ethical principles in resolving medical ethics problems. Additional rules, or guidelines for relating theory and practice, must be developed according to this approach. Among these rules is the context functioning as a formal adjustment to values in concrete circumstances. Earlier I emphasized the importance of consideration of the particularities of a case, including its context, for a properly compassionate analysis.

The root of the difficulty in medical ethics lies in a confrontation between an abstracting tendency in the long and rewarding history of ethics and the concrete, individual problems encountered by professionals. The latter must make quick decisions about very complex matters in order to benefit their patients. Contrariwise, ethical analysis must take careful note of numerous ethical theories, axioms, and other concerns in order to conduct a minimally decent conceptual and problematical analysis. This process takes time and, of necessity, becomes quite abstract. Health professionals and patients quickly lose interest in these abstractions and theoretical meanderings if they are not decisively and explicitly related to the realities of patient care. They must do ethics on the run.

Ethical principles appear abstract—or better, speculative—because they do not possess the same degree of social legitimacy as the values of everyday life. Moral abstractions frequently are seen by non-philosophers as empty of the normal ingredients of moral concerns people have in their day-to-day life. No doubt they can and do seep into that daily life, but the process of connecting theory to practice is a long and subtle one in most cases.[35] How often do we encounter physicians and patients who become impatient with "thinking" that has no practical consequence.

Thus, according to the contextualism theory, what is needed is a means by which to locate a moral problem and to exhibit the likely values and principles at issue within that locus. The context having been established by such a "grid," the discussion can proceed toward means for resolving the case by protecting the interests and values of those affected by it. But that is not all. The grid not only locates and focuses the moral discussion, it also hints at the cross-case commonalities that legitimize the very act of organizing similar cases, comparing them, and drawing conclusions about the new case.

There is a variability of contexts in the clinical resolution of cases that is noticeable to all who work in the medical setting. This variability does not describe so much the relativity of values and principles; rather, it describes how the weight they bring to bear on a case is partially determined by the medical specialty involved, the personal values of the patient, family, or social group, the personal and professional values of the health care professionals involved, and the institutional setting in which the problem arises. Some principles and axioms will be given more weight than others in such a scheme, and one important component of the weighting will stem from the contexts. The good will arise out of the mix of these components.

Such a contextual grid is only one aspect, then, of what might be called context-variable moral rules. Other examples could be examined that do not fit the contextual grid pattern, but are moral rules which in other ways vary with the context. Further, the contextual grid I propose cannot encompass all of the variables in a case—but only the ones most likely to be affecting the emphasis of some values or principles over others. This is precisely where deductive models of ethical reasoning fall short.

An example follows: the rule of protection of autonomy is more likely to be given prominent focus in a primary care context than in a tertiary care one, wherein one's autonomy is virtually always depressed and hence concern for autonomy is diminished in favor of a goal of preservation of life and/or restoration of health.[36] Furthermore, the rule of protection of autonomy is more likely to be emphasized in cases in which there is no threat to others than in cases wherein the common good must be considered, sometimes to the detriment of personal autonomy. Finally, because the grid only *describes* most likely weights given to moral principles and rules in formulating an indicated course of action, one should not misconstrue the contextual grid as claiming that physicians in tertiary care settings do not care about protecting their patients' autonomy, or that public health officials stress social responsibility to the exclusion of individual well-being. All of these moral values bear upon a case. The grid only describes what values are most likely to take precedence over others.

The contextual grid theory rests on two distinctions. The first is the distinction between primary, secondary, and tertiary care settings, a standard distinction in medicine. This distinction forms one set of coordinates of the grid. Its importance for moral reasoning lies in the seriousness of the assault on personal wholeness brought about by the disease in question.[37] Thus, a patient's wishes are more likely to be sought and respected in a primary care setting than in an emergency room after a heart attack, where a paternalistic response may be, and often is, more appropriate. The second distinction or coordinate of the grid is that between the individual and the number of persons affected by the problem. The moral significance of this distinction is based on the increasing complexity of values the more different persons whose interests are affected by the outcome of the case enter our consideration, and our increased tendency to protect the commonweal the greater the number of affected persons. Recall again the purpose of the grid is to describe context-variable rules, i.e., which principles and axioms are likely to be given more weight than others in a given circumstance in formulating a moral policy or in developing an indicated course of action.

Compassionate Analysis

Advances have occurred in emphasizing not only the rights of patients to determine the treatments they desire and do not desire during the dying process, but also the development of the rights to choose treatments at any time during life, not just while dying. The efforts of patient advocacy groups in sponsoring and supporting legislation and court deliberations have been outstanding. The Living Will and Advance Directives, including the Durable Power of Attorney, all point to eventual further clarification of these rights, for example, how they will have an impact on long-term care settings.[38] What is important to note is that the underlying motivation for the development of such instruments is the prevention of suffering, that is, to increase the role of compassion in decisions about life-prolonging technology.[39,40] It would make sense to extend these rights to even greater control over the dying process.

As noted earlier, medical technology gives us enormous power at all levels of life, but especially at the end of life. Yet concerns should not be confined to dispatching persons too early by injections in active, direct euthanasia, while not meeting their physical and social needs. Another form of the "technofix" society is to prolong suffering in conditions of hopeless injury to life. "Hopeless injury" as Braithwaite and I defined it is:

> a condition in which there is no potential for growth or repair; no observable pleasure or happiness from living . . . and a total absence of one or more of the following attributes of quality of life: cognition or recognition, motor activity, memory or awareness of time, consciousness, and language or other intelligent means of communicating thoughts or wishes.[41]

Daily life is full of interactions with "things"—nonhuman and fundamentally incomprehensible to most persons. We sometimes get so used to technological processes that we behave as though they are substitutes for human and compassionate care. Eating for many elderly and dying patients has been replaced by tubes; participating in the spiritual and material values of human life has been replaced by "merely surviving," as a being subjugated to the very products of human imagination. As Illich observes:

> Medical civilization is planned and organized to kill pain, to eliminate sickness, and to abolish the need for acts of suffering and dying[42] . . .
> The new experience that has replaced dignified suffering is artificially prolonged, opaque, depersonalized maintenance.[43]

Such "beings" on depersonalized maintenance may no longer be as human as the rest of us, precisely because of this subjugation. This is no way to respect the value of human life. Is a permanently unconscious being without any ability to relate to its environment a "person?" Part of taking responsibility for our technology is to avoid this subjugation of human life to machinery in the first place, through more thorough discussions of possible outcomes and patient values regarding them.

Compassionate contextualism has the following features:

1. Just as in aesthetics, one must know both the whole and the individual parts. Moral reasoning from both rationalistic and emotional openness means that the "big picture" is combined with the sophisticated understanding of the individual's plight, values, and possible outcomes. One is neither unduly swayed by reason or emotion, but by a balance between the two.

    A good example might be a case in which a fourteen-year-old child rejects a blood transfusion for religious reasons. She and her mother are recent converts to the Jehovah's Witnesses faith. She is the only surviving individual on an initial remission cancer protocol, but now suffers from *Pneumocystis carinii* pneumonia. Her compromised immunological state with few white blood cells remaining means that, without a transfusion, she will die. She does not want to die, but she does want to be true to her fundamental religious principles. To complicate matters, her mother and she are converts based on the religion of her mother's third husband. She has changed religion with each marriage. The mother has a history of instability.

An clinical ethicist, unfamiliar with all the ramifications of the case, might argue on rational grounds that society grants power to pediatricians to protect the lives of such children. In some states, doctors have forty-eight hours during which they are to take over the case to protect the child while they seek a court order for custodial decision making on behalf of the child. Yet a more complete understanding of the case includes an awareness of the girl's valiant fight against cancer, her maturity beyond her years, the strength of her own religious convictions, the bonds of love between the mother and child, and their sense of belonging to a religious community. All of these might be shattered in a decision to override her wishes and give her the transfusion. The latter may not be successful in any case.

2. The life of the patient has a certain "completeness" about it that transcends reason. It is discerned instinctively by the caregivers and surrogates. This "completeness" or wholeness of a life leads to decisions in some instances that might not otherwise be rationally defensible.

Consider the case of a nurse, daughter of a veterinarian and nurse, and eldest sister of three nurses. The youngest sister was driving a car, making a left turn, when the car was broadsided. The patient's head was broken from her spine at C2, and held on the body only by the muscle tissue of the neck. After stabilization it was determined that, although not brain-dead, significant damage had occurred to her brain. Even if she were to live, she would be in a permanent vegetative state and permanently paralyzed. Her parents, opening an ethics consult meeting with a prayer, tearfully expressed her view that she wanted to donate her organs. It became evident to everyone at the meeting, the hospital administrator, the neurologists, the chaplain, the nurses, and the ethicist, that her life would not acquire its divine completeness without donation of her organs. Her parents argued very successfully, not only through reasonable statements, but also through their grief, that this and only this would give meaning to their daughter's commitment to care for others, and help them cope with her death. All of us agreed that she should have her organs taken prior to removing her from life-support systems.

This decision, important as it was, violated the law. The law requires that individuals be brain-dead before donation occurs. In her case, withdrawing life-support would contribute to the dying of the organs as well. The transplant team, a different group than that which met with the family during the ethics consult, refused to accept the decision on legal grounds, fearing they might be contributing to the death rather than taking the organs after a legal death had been proclaimed.

This case changed the way I think about organ donation, and led to a chapter I wrote arguing in favor of organ donation in a permanent vegetative state as well as when one is brain-dead.[44]

3. The grounds for the decision are not ultimately made on the basis of current practice, although these principles are important, but on the basis of helping the person complete their life. In a spy novel by John Le Carré, *The Secret Pilgrim*, George Smiley says: "The purpose of *my* life was to end the time I lived in."[45] This statement gains particular poignancy when individuals combine reasons with compassion in dealing with issues at the end of life.

CONCLUSION

In a society such as ours, with its problems of poverty, homelessness, gaining access to health care, and denigration of the weak, we need to maintain constant vigilance about protecting persons from both undertreatment and abandonment and inappropriate overtreatment. In both instances, we will be shepherding our technology to good human aims. This is compassion.

NOTES

1. Jonsen, A., "Casuistry as Methodology in Clinical Ethics," *Theoretical Medicine* 1992;12:295–308.

2. Jonsen, A., Toulmin, S., *The Abuse of Casuistry: A History of Moral Reasoning* (Berkeley, CA: University of California Press, 1988).

3. Tomlinson, T., "Casuistry in Medical Ethics: Rehabilitated or Repeat Offender?" *Theoretical Medicine* 1994;15: in press.

4. Pellegrino, E. D., Thomasma, D. C., *A Philosophical Basis of Medical Practice* (New York: Oxford University Press, 1981).

5. Bruce Buursma, "Pollster Gallup Feels Spirit Traveling All Over the World," *Chicago Tribune* Friday, August 1, 1986, Sect. 2, 7, quotes Gallup as observing that there is a major shift worldwide "away from all forms of anti-religion and nonreligious ideology." "People in many nations appear to be searching with a new intensity for spiritual moorings."

However, this search has been accompanied by a decline in morality. This paradox Gallup has charted in the United States, and it is now found all around the world. In short, while an increase in spiritual yearning has occurred, a corresponding decrease in belief in a God who cares about human life, and to whom individuals are accountable, has also occurred. Gallup believes, however, that the search for meaning can be translated into real faith and action for many people.

6. MacIntyre, A., *After Virtue*, 2d ed. (Notre Dame, IN: University of Notre Dame Press, 1984).

7. Jonsen, A., What Does Life Support Support? in Winslade, W., ed., *Personal Choices and Public Commitments: Perspectives on the Humanities* (Galveston, TX: Institute for the Medical Humanities, 1988:61–69), quote:66–67.

8. Raffin, T. A., Shurkin, J. N., Sinkler, W. III, *Intensive Care: Facing the Critical Issues* (New York: W. H. Freeman & Co., 1988), 185.

9. Ibid, 175.

10. Scitovsky, A. A., Capron, A. M., "Medical Care at the End of Life: The Interaction of Economics and Ethics," *Ann. Revue of Public Health* 1986; 7:59–75.

11. Bernadin, J., Euthanasia: Ethical and Legal Challenge. Address to the Center for Clinical Medical Ethics, University of Chicago Hospital, May 26, 1988, 16.

12. Bernadin, 14.

13. Pellegrino, E. D., and Thomasma, D. C., *The Christian Virtues in Medicine*. (Washington, DC: Georgetown University Press, in press).

14. Pellegrino, E. D., Thomasma, D. C., *For the Patient's Good: The Restoration of Beneficence in Health Care* (New York: Oxford University Press, 1988).

15. Loewy, E., "The Restoration of Beneficence," *Hastings Center Report* 1989;19:42–43.

16. Engelhardt, H. T., Jr., *Bioethics and Secular Humanism* (London/Philadelphia, PA: SCM/Trinity Press International, 1991).

17. Blum, L., "Moral Perception and Particularity," *Ethics* 1991;101:701–725.

18. Walker, M. U., "Moral Particularity," *Metaphilosophy* 1987;18, nos. 3 and 4:171–185.

19. Franklin, B., *Franklin: The Autobiography* (New York: Vintage Books/The Library of America, 1990), p. 55.

20. Gaylin, W., Kass, L., Pellegrino, E. D., Siegler, M., "Commentaries: Doctors Must Not Kill." *J American Medical Association* 1988;259:2139–40.

21. Kass, L., "Arguments against Active Euthanasia by Doctors Found at Medicine's Core," *Kennedy Institute of Ethics Newsletter* Jan 1989;3:1–3,6.

22. Pope John Paul II, *Humanize Hospital Work*, Address to the Sixty-First General Chapter of the Hospital Order of St. John of God. *L'Osservatore Romano*, January 24, 1983:3.

23. Flannery, A., *Vatican II: The Conciliar and Post-Conciliar Documents* (Collegeville MN: Liturgical Press, 1975), Decree on the Apostolate of the Laity.

24. Nouwen, H., *The Wounded Healer* (New York: Doubleday, 1972):72.

25. De Unamuno, M., *The Tragic Sense of Life* (Princeton: Bollingen Series, LXXXV, 4; 1972), translated by Anthony Kerrigan:224.

26. Pope John Paul II, *Rich in Mercy* (the Encyclical *Dives in Misericordia*), November 30, 1980 (Washington, DC: U.S. Catholic Conference, 1981): 45.

27. Bergsma, J., and Thomasma, D. C., *Health Care: Its Psychosocial Dimensions* (Pittsburgh, PA: Duquesne University Press, 1983).

28. Pellegrino, E. D., and Thomasma, D. C., *Health and Healing* (published in an Italian translation first), (Rome: Editions Deshoines, in press).

29. Pellegrino, E. D., Thomasma, D. C., *The Virtues in Medical Practice* (New York: Oxford University Press, 1993).

30. Ibid.

31. Pope John Paul II, *Rich in Mercy,* 46.

32. Jonsen, A., Toulmin, S., *The Abuse of Casuistry.*

33. McIntyre, A., *After Virtue.*

34. Thomasma, D., "The Context as Moral Rule in Medical Ethics," *J Bioethics* 1984;5:63–79.

35. Graber, G. C., and Thomasma, D. C., *Theory and Practice in Medical Ethics* (New York: Continuum, 1989).

36. Thomasma, D.C., "Beyond Medical Paternalism and Patient Autonomy: A Model of Physician's Conscience for the Doctor-Patient Relationship," *Ann Internal Medicine* 1983;98:243-248.

37. Bergsma, J., Thomasma, D.C., *Health Care.*

38. Rouse, F., "Living Wills in the Long-term Care Setting." *J Long-Term Care Administration* 1988;17:14–19.

39. Mehling, A., "Living Wills: Preventing Suffering or a Deadly Contract?" *State Government News* Dec 1988:14–15.

40. Mehling, A., Neitlich, S., "Right-to-die Backgrounder," *News from the Society for the Right to Die* (Now Choice in Dying), January 1989:1–2.

41. Braithwaite, S., Thomasma, D. C., "New Guidelines on Foregoing Life-sustaining Treatment in Incompetent Patients: An Anti-cruelty Policy," *Ann Internal Medicine* 1986;104:711–15.

42. Illich, I., *Medical Nemesis: The Expropriation of Health* (New York: Pantheon, 1976):106.

43. Ibid, 154.

44. Thomasma, D. C., "Making Treatment Decisions for Permanently Unconscious Patients: The Ethical Perspective," in John F. Monagle and David C. Thomasma, eds., *Medical Ethics: A Guide for Health Professionals* (Rockville, MD: Aspen Publishers, 1988):192–204.

45. John Le Carré, *The Secret Pilgrim* (New York: Alfred Knopf, 1991), 12.

NARRATIVE:

Beyond the Clinical Gaze

W. Thomas Boyce

The late French philosopher and sociologist Michel Foucault argued in his book *The Birth of the Clinic* (London: Tavistock, 1973) that the *gaze* (or vision) of Western medicine was fundamentally transformed in the eighteenth century by the advent of the autopsy. For the first time in the history of medicine, physicians were invited to peer into the darkened recesses of the human body and find there the locus, the very substance, of disease. Foucault observed that this revolutionary change— the capacity for gazing upon and touching the lesions that are the sources of infirmity and death—altered forever our ways of *seeing* patients and their afflictions. From that time forward human illness became embodied within the pathological material of the disease process, and the search for lesions—be they tumors or pathogens or disordered genomes—became the principal and essential business of medical care.

The products of this changed vision, this new way of seeing and interpreting the signposts of disease, are abundant and all about us. Fiber optic endoscopes place our eyes at the threshold of a duodenal ulcer. Magnetic resonance images allow both physician and patient to visualize a malignancy deep within the midbrain. Electron microscopy brings into view the pathological changes, measured in microns, in the kidney tubules of a nephrotic child. For those of us who frequent and inhabit the "cathedrals" of modern medicine, there is, I think, a kind of dazzling euphoria to be found in our seemingly endless capacity for seeing deeper, better, and more penetratingly into the heart of disease.

And, yet, for many of us, there is a suspicion, a gnawing discomfort about the splendid technological extensions of the medical gaze that changed so dramatically three centuries ago. For me, there is a growing unease that, in our headlong efforts to bring into focus finer and more discriminating views of the lesions lying *beneath* disease, we

144

will have missed the opportunity to envision the person or the patient that lies *beyond* the disease. In my life as a pediatrician, this discomfort has become what I would characterize as the ethical or philosophical equivalent of a prolonged headache: a constant backdrop of low-grade pain, a touch of vaguely nauseating concern over how serious its etiology might be, and an awareness of something not quite right in my base of operations.

A little more than a year ago during my month serving as the attending physician on the pediatrics ward of the University of California, San Francisco, I ran across a dying boy who, together with his mother, reminded me, as I often am reminded, of the troubled, myopic vision so characteristic of the medicine I have learned and practice. He was a relatively young boy (I will call him Blake), no more than seven years of age and afflicted with a terminal, disfiguring version of mucolipidosis. For those unfamiliar with this disorder, it is a genetically based storage disease involving the pathological accumulation of complex carbohydrates in many tissues of the body, including the bones and joints, the heart, eyes, liver, spleen, and brain. It is a disease that is slowly progressive, usually ending in death from heart or lung failure within the first decade of life.

Over the years of Blake's short life, the unabated metabolic hoarding of carbohydrates had severely deformed and retarded him. His eyes were clouded and protruded from his face as did his tongue, like the overstuffed contents of a pastry shell too small to contain it. The gums surrounding his peg-like teeth were similarly engorged and frequently bled when disturbed. His massively swollen heart was failing, and he perenially threatened to drown in the secretions that flooded his airway. His chest and belly, glutted with a liver and spleen many times their normal sizes, had together become a single, reddened, congested globe from which four largely useless limbs projected. He was, in short, a small, grotesque tomato-of-a-boy whose appearance turned away even the most forgiving eyes.

Blake also was not overly grateful for the abundant, cutting edge medical care being provided for him. I think he somehow sensed that he was nearing the end of his time, and he had decided that the sticks and pokes and serial examinations did almost nothing to allay the other torments that his disease had long prolonged. So, the approach of doctors, nurses, technicians, and all the other assorted hospital personnel was greeted abruptly with a raspy incoherent grunt and a flailing motion of his arm that meant, indisputably, "Get out of my face!"

Blake's intolerance for the hospital and its staff, together with his unsavory countenance, made him a difficult patient for whom to care. His medical "care" was difficult by virtue of his resistance to our routines and procedures. But my own ability to humanly care for Blake also was compromised by the physical sight of him and by his stolid indifference or antagonism to my best efforts on his behalf.

One July evening, held in the hospital late by a series of unanticipated events, I approached Blake's room at an unaccustomed hour. His young, single mom, who was at her own place of work for the daylight hours of most days, was sitting on the edge of the bed, deeply immersed in a conversation with Blake. I paused, and then settled at the door, transfixed by the scene before me in the darkened hospital room. Blake's mom was talking to him. In hushed and comforting tones she spoke of the day, wondering how things had gone, asking him about his new nurse, reviewing for him the events of her own day at work. As she spoke, leaning over her son, her hand stroked his forehead and hair in a mundane gesture that filled the room with her love for the boy.

Blake's eyes, moist and utterly devoid of his stern resistance, looked up into his mother's face, absorbing every moment, every piece of her presence there with him. Relaxed and more peaceful than I had ever seen him, Blake seemed to melt into his mother's eyes. She stroked his round, swollen face and said to him, "Oh, my beautiful, little boy."

Suddenly I understood what I had not understood: When this mother gazed at her bloated, dying son, she *physically saw* a person I had never seen. Transformed by her eyes' willingness to see the child *beyond* the disease, Blake had become a different being, an individual no longer diseased and distorted, but a frightened child visibly changed by his mother's love.

In the months since that night and since his death later in that same year, I often have thought of Blake and his mother. I have thought of how limited my vision of my patients has been, of the peculiar and short-sighted lenses through which so much of our vaunted medicine is conducted. I have thought of how mysteriously my own way of seeing Blake was irreparably changed by the experience of watching his mom truly see him and respond to him for who he, finally, was.

I have thought, as well, of Jesus and the clarity of his sight: his capacity for seeing through all the littered crustiness of a person's life into the heart of an individual soul. I have remembered Jesus' encounter with the Samaritan woman at Jacob's well and how terrifyingly he took in and captured the totality of that woman's failed life. And, seeing the depth of her need and the desperation in her hidden thirst for the substance of life, he offered her living water, promising that whoever drinks of the water he provides will find an everlasting spring and a source of eternal life. Imagine the transformation that Samaritan woman must have experienced two thousand years ago! How the clarity of Christ's gaze, burning like a refiner's fire, reduced all of the complexity, ambiguity, and uncertainty of her broken past into a single vision of her greatest need, and then answered that need thoroughly and unconditionally.

I have been looked upon by the eyes of Jesus. At a time of extraordinary despair, so extraordinary that even now it is difficult to look back on it, I was gazed upon and touched by the presence of Christ in the most mundane of settings, at the most unexpected of times. Overwhelmed in those days with a crushing, killing vision of my own inadequacy for life, I found myself utterly surrounded, for a moment no longer than Blake's conversation with his mom, by the palpable, unmistakable, and overpowering presence of God's love.

In that moment, now many years ago, it was clear to me that I was seen for who I was and am. And that I was changed forever by the Lord's willingness to look on me and find in me a creature worthy of his love and care.

The wonder of Jesus' way of seeing people, such as me and Blake and countless others, is that it is a *transforming* vision. It is an instrumental vision that reaches into the essential character of the person and alters that character at its core. It is, miraculously, a way of seeing that is accessible to all of us and one that transforms not only the person seen, but also the person seeing.

In his book *Life on the Mississippi*, Mark Twain wrote of the grief and disappointment he experienced as a steamboat captain's apprentice one summer in his youth. Learning to navigate the Mississippi's currents and memorizing in great detail the visible signs of its topography and course, he noted how the mystery and awe of that great river began to recede from his youthful grasp and how the river itself seemed changed. "Since that time," he wrote, "I have pitied doctors from my heart. . . . Does [the doctor] ever again see [a young child's] beauty . . . or doesn't he simply view her professionally, and comment upon her unwholesome condition all to himself? And doesn't he sometimes wonder whether he has gained most or lost most by learning his trade" (in *The Family Mark Twain*, New York: Barnes and Noble, [1883] 1992, p. 47).

He wonders indeed. He wonders, as I suspect we all must wonder, about what has been lost in the learning of our various disciplines, in the developing of our various ways of seeing the patients and clients who come to us bearing their all too visible frailties. But there is in the vision of Christ, even in the vision of Blake's mother, a redemptive view in which all of the wonder, hope, and humanity that each of our patients bears along to us is not lost, but is seen. In that seeing there is a hope, I believe, for a better medicine. A *new* medicine that, along with all the helping professions, reaffirms that call for a clearer vision of the business of caring, and for new eyes and new ways of seeing.

Caring as Gift and Goal: Biblical and Theological Reflections

JOEL B. GREEN

INTRODUCTION

As a lexeme, "caring" is not particularly theological or biblical; one looks in vain for it in the standard reference works. "Caring" nevertheless evokes a wide range of concepts—especially those terms related to the semantic fields of mercy and justice—and these occupy a central place both in the biblical witness and in theological reflection. A closely related set of terms, terms with profound interpersonal and systemic implications that figure prominently in the message of Jesus, embraces the concept of servanthood. The Evangelist Luke reports Jesus' programmatic words on this subject:

> The rulers of the non-Jewish people exercise lordship over them, and those with authority are treated with special honor. Let it not be so with you! Rather, let the greatest among you be as the youngest, the leader as one who serves.[1]

As prominent as this concern might have been for Jesus and the early Jesus-movement, the sort of "service" for which Jesus called and which he himself demonstrated, was not eagerly sanctioned in first-century Roman antiquity. Nor is this term easily embraced in late-twentieth-century North America. If, as Suzanne Gordon suggests,[2] "caring" has fallen on hard times because of its popular association with codependency, so that people can "love too much" and "caring" can be interpreted as a symptom leading to the diagnosis of psychosocial maladjustment, then the modern connotations of "servanthood" are even more negative.

Unfortunately, it is not because it presents a countercultural alternative to society-at-large that the concept of "servanthood" has

149

been held at arm's length in recent times. This was certainly the case
in Jesus' day, but no longer in ours. Indeed, it is arguable that
"servant-hood" has become too much a term in the service of dominant culture today. Herein lies the scandal: It is precisely as this term
has been (mis)interpreted and (mis)applied by and within communities of Christian faith that the negative nuances of "service" have
developed and disseminated widely both within and outside the
church. The church's record vis-à-vis women (and especially married
women) is only one highly visible case in point, for the phenomenon
of encouraging others to docile subjection, submission, and positions
of shameful status with appeal to the words and example of Jesus is
widespread. This is not to suggest that "following the example of
Jesus" should no longer be in fashion today; the challenge of the *imitatio Christi* has a long and significant record in Christian history, evident in a profound way already in 1 Peter.[3] Rather, it is a recognition
that "serving" today, and with it "caring," has become in many circles
yet one more weapon in the arsenal of the control-oriented paradigm.
The challenge to service is often heard as the command, "Serve me!"
or "Serve our institution (including the church-as-institution)!" One is
reminded of the self-serving abuses of some itinerant prophets
already in the first century, who turned their offices and gifts into
exploitative opportunities, which led to the instruction,

> Let every apostle who comes to your home be received as you
> would receive the Lord. But do not let your visitor stay longer
> than a day—or perhaps two, if need be. Whoever stays three
> days is a false prophet. . . . And no prophet who orders a meal
> while caught up in the spirit shall eat of that meal; whoever
> does so is a false prophet.[4]

It may be that the remedy needed involves adopting a new set of
terms, symbols devoid of the negative connotations that we now find
so interwoven with these significant words. What, then, will protect
those words from misapplication, unless the stories behind the words
themselves are spoken again in our consciousness? In the story of
God's engagement with God's people, how did these concepts arise?
What did they mean? Such queries as these set the agenda for this
essay. Rather than work our way through the whole of the biblical
materials, a task whose proportions far outstrip our needs, we will
focus attention in the first instance on a theme central to theological

anthropology—namely, the *imago Dei*, the affirmation that human beings are made in God's own image. Here, in this concept, are the foundational bearings for developing a theological perspective on human interaction in general and caring in particular. Having briefly explored the meaning of this phrase, we will see how the *imago Dei* has been foundational to ethical comportment in the Scriptures of Israel and in the New Testament. Finally, we will go on to develop a portrait of service from the Fourth Gospel, showing in a further way how caring and service are deeply rooted in the bedrock of Christian faith.

THE *IMAGO DEI*

For persons who take seriously the contours of the way the biblical books themselves handle the theological task, faith and praxis must arise out of the community's understanding and experience of God. Scripture simply knows no detached or abstract theology, no speculation about the nature of God in Himself or about the nature of humanity in itself. Affirmations of "the eternal character of God," for example, appear in the Book of Revelation ("him who is, who was, and who is to come . . . the Alpha and the Omega"),[5] but not as a manifestation of disengaged theology; rather, in the context of grave distress at the end of the first century, the Christian community in Asia Minor, John deemed, needed a reminder that *God was God* before the appearance of the current crisis, *God will be God* when the present world situation will have been transformed, and *God is God* even in the midst of this trauma. It is no surprise, then, that a theological understanding of caring will take as its primary point of departure the nature of God particularly in relation to God's purposeful engagement with the world.

The Story of Creation

From the standpoint of the biblical canon, the starting point is the story of creation, particularly the creation of humanity. The opening chapter of the Book of Genesis focuses initially on the nonhuman creation. It is created first, has its own relation to God, and receives divine blessing. Nevertheless, the staging of the chapter places special emphasis on the creation of humanity:

> Then God said, "Let us make humanity in our image, after our own likeness. Let them have dominion over the fish of the sea,

over the birds of the air, over the cattle, over the whole earth, and over every creeping thing that creeps upon the earth." So God created humanity in his own image, in the image of God he created them; male and female he created them. And God blessed them, and said to them, "Be fruitful and multiply, and fill the earth and subdue it. Have dominion over the fish of the sea, the birds of the air, and over every living thing that moves upon the earth."[6]

Of all the creatures mentioned in this story, only humanity is created after God's own likeness, in God's own image. Only to humanity does God speak directly. Humanity alone receives from God a divine vocation. In creation, God shapes a covenant relationship with all creatures, but among these the God-human relationship is extraordinary.

What is meant by the *imago Dei*? Although the biblical text affirms clearly *that* humans are created in God's image, it is not entirely clear regarding *what* this entails. As a result, throughout the history of Christianity it has received a diversity of interpretations.[7] No one holds today, as some did earlier, that the *imago Dei* refers to some physical characteristic of humanity, such as standing upright. A number of theologians have found the key to this concept in the reasoning powers of human beings, especially (as in Augustine) the human capacity to know God. Others have pointed to the human conscience or more generally to the moral responsibility of humanity. Still others have queried whether the divine image can be located in any particular, static quality or capacity of human beings.

Taken within its immediate narrative co-text in Genesis 1, "the image of God" in which humanity is made transparently relates to the exercise of dominion over the earth on God's behalf. But this only begs the question, for we must then ascertain what it means to exercise dominion in this way—that is, in a way that reflects God's own style of interaction with his creatures. What is more, this way of putting the issue does not grapple with the profound word spoken over humanity and about humanity, that human beings in themselves (and not only in what they do) reflect the divine image.

On such matters, Karl Barth has proven particularly insightful.[8] For him, creation is the external basis of the covenant (which relationship itself grows out of God's own character), for in humanity God created for himself a counterpart, a covenant partner.

> For the meaning and purpose of God at his creation were as fol-
> lows. He willed the existence of a being which in all its non-
> deity and therefore its differentiation can be a real partner;
> which is capable of action and responsibility in relation to Him;
> to which His own divine form of life is not alien; which in a crea-
> turely repetition, as a copy and imitation, can be a bearer of this
> form of life. Man [sic] was created as this being. But the divine
> form of life, repeated in the man created by Him, consists in that
> which is the obvious aim of the "Let us." In God's own being
> and sphere there is a counterpart: a genuine but harmonious self-
> encounter and self-discovery; a free co-existence and co-opera-
> tion; an open confrontation and reciprocity.[9]

Barth's understanding of the *imago Dei* is particularly Christian in the
way it focuses attention on the phrase, "Let *us* make humanity in *our*
own image." Barth finds in this "us" and "our" the community of the
Godhead, so that any reflection of God's image would of necessity
have a communal orientation.[10] From this, human beings draw their
affirmation of exalted worth and reason for being, their fundamental
vocation. Thus, humanity is created in relationship to God and finds
itself as a result of its creation in covenant with God. And humanity is
given the divine mandate to reflect God's own covenant love in relation with God, with the covenant community of all humanity, and
with all that God has created.

   It is true that the vocabulary of the creation story has led some
to take a disparaging attitude toward and grossly to abuse nature.
After all, the imperatives "exercise dominion" and "subdue" seem far
removed from notions of care and covenant love. Such understanding
and behavior have no basis here, however. First, inasmuch as these
responsibilities are rooted in the shaping of humans *in God's image*,
human dominion must reflect God's own rule of the world and there
is no notion here of coercive or tyrannical power. Second, the terminology itself suggests other connotations within the biblical tradition—e.g., where "ruling" is the act of the shepherd who provides for,
cares for the flock. As Walter Brueggemann remarks, "[T]he task of
'dominion' does not have to do with exploitation or abuse. It has to
do with securing the well-being of every other creature and bringing
the promise of each to full fruition."[11]

   This reminder has implications for caring among humans as
well, for it suggests what sort of behavior on behalf of others is

worthy of being described as "caring." Brueggemann's language about securing the well-being of every other creature and bringing the promise of each to full fruition extends as well to caring human interaction. "Caregiving" is in fact "caring" when it empowers and frees care receivers to fulfill their divine vocation as members of the human family. "Caregiving" in this sense does not arise from any interest in controlling the attitudes or behaviors of others, or predetermining the consequences of those actions, nor primarily from a sense of obligation. Caregiving that takes its bearings from the character of God expressed in creation grows out of one's own interested love and concern for human wholeness.

From a theological standpoint, any notions of caring we might have grow out of this divine vocation, to reflect in our lives together in the world the character of God manifest in his covenant love. By "covenant love" we mean the compassionate behavior of God that issues in the formation of covenant relationship with human beings, not behavior that derives from a previously established covenant. Covenant love is not loyalty, but surprising, gracious care that goes beyond expected norms of mutual obligation. This is the compassion of God manifest in creation. Humanity is the recipient of this covenant love, but as bearers of the divine image, human beings are also recipients of the capacity themselves "to do" covenant love. This is God's gift to humanity, but it is also the goal of human interaction.[12] Thus: In creation, God endows humanity with the capacity and the vocation to engage in gracious relationship with Himself; in creation, God endows humanity with the capacity and the vocation to engage in gracious relationship with their fellow human beings; in creation, God endows humanity with the capacity and the vocation to engage in relationship with all creation. To be in gracious relationship, to care, is to reflect the divine image. It is to be human.

Exodus and the New Community

According to the Genesis narrative, in spite of the continued refusal to fulfill their vocation and reflect in their lives together the divine image, men and women continued to be the object of God's focused care. In the sense just outlined, people did not want to be human; they rejected their status as finite creatures who "find themselves" always in relation to God, the larger human community, and all creation. Nevertheless, repeatedly, and through a variety of people, God continued to initiate gracious interaction with humanity. As the Book of Genesis closes and the Book of Exodus opens, the spotlight has fallen on the descendants of Jacob, who now find themselves in Egypt in an oppressed state. Deuteronomy 26:5–9, regarded by many scholars as an early, narratological "confession of faith," outlines the story as it now develops:

> A wandering Aramean was my ancestor; he went down into Egypt and lived there as a stranger, few in number, and there he became a great nation, mighty and large in number. Then the Egyptians oppressed us by imposing hard labor on us, and we cried out to the Lord, the God of our ancestors. The Lord heard our voice, saw our affliction, toil, and oppression. The Lord brought us out of Egypt with a mighty hand and outstretched arm, with a terrifying display of power, and with signs and wonders. He brought us to this place; he gave us this land, a land flowing with milk and honey.

Here are summarized the seminal events at the root of Israel's self-understanding as God's people. God had looked graciously upon them in their distress and had taken away their oppression. Fundamental to this act of God was His taking their side, the side of those living on the margins of Egyptian society. Just as critical, however, was *the way* God chose to rescue Israel, not by bringing reform within their oppressed contexts but by transplanting them to a new setting. In doing so, He created a new people, a new nation.[13] And a chief characteristic of this new nation was that it would be a people among whom oppression was absent. It is in this context that we must understand the giving of the law.

Since the days of Martin Luther in the sixteenth century, it has been widely assumed that, into a Judaism characterized by legalistic adherence to the law, first Jesus, then Paul came with a message of grace. *They* were burdened by the law and worked night and day to achieve some glimmer of God's grace; in Christ, *we* have become the recipients of unmerited love. It now appears that this unfortunate way of putting things grew out of a highly contextualized reading of the New Testament on the part of Luther. He understood the church of his day to be overly concerned with how one might "work one's way" into friendship with God; he rediscovered the message that God extends friendship as the first act—that a new relationship with God depended on God's grace, to which humans are called to respond in faith. The mistake has been our continued retroversion of Luther's interpretation of his sociohistorical situation in the sixteenth century back into Paul's and Jesus' settings in the first. In fact, the central claim of the Jewish people in the first century clearly related to their standing as God's covenant people. Had not God chosen them and delivered them out of Egypt?

In other words, the giving of the law was not the institution of a legalism. The giving of the law was not God's way of keeping these previously marginalized people "in line." Seen within the context of God's gracious act of deliverance and creation of this new people in the exodus experience, the giving of the law must be understood as a concrete embodiment of God's own character within this new community. Israel must not be like Egypt, taking advantage of the vulnerable people of its society; rather, God's people are to reflect within their lives together God's own concern for the "little people."

This reality is seen in myriads of ways in the Books of Exodus, Leviticus, Numbers, and Deuteronomy, often in the way the many regulations are spelled out. For example,

> When you reap your harvest in your field and forget a sheaf in the field, you shall not go back to get it; it shall be left for the alien, the orphan, and the widow, so that the Lord your God may bless you in all your undertakings. When you beat your olive trees, do not strip what is left; it shall be left for the alien, the orphan, and the widow. When you gather the grapes of your vineyard, do not glean what is left; it shall be left for the alien, the orphan, and the widow. Remember that you were a slave in the land of Egypt; therefore I am commanding you to do this.[14]

This text is particularly instructive because of its repeated concern for the alien, the orphan, and the widow—who together made up a class of expendable people. The final sentence, "Remember that you were a slave in the land of Egypt," serves to draw a direct parallel between these expendables in Israelite society and Israel itself in Egyptian society. Just as God was concerned for Israel in its distress, so God is concerned for these little people in theirs. As God demonstrated His care for Israel in the exodus, so Israel shall care for these little people. In this way they embody God's own character.

Although scarcely absent in earlier biblical material, the election of Israel and gift of the law are also the occasion for a renewed and explicit emphasis on the spirituality that drives human behavior in community and world. Human interaction and social dynamics are to grow out of a profound understanding and experience of God and His covenant love. Central to Israel's spirituality would be the *Shema*—"Hear, O Israel: The Lord our God is one Lord," from which flows the admonition to love God with heart, soul, and strength.[15] Set within the larger framework of the commandments of God ordering Israel's common life, this call is a profound affirmation that ethical comportment grows out of the friendships and practices of a community oriented around the redeeming God.

The law, then, was not given as a canon for measuring the relative holiness of a people. The law was grace, an invitation to redemptive relationship; the law gave expression to the character of the community God had called, setting before God's people the nature of the community to which they were called. Here was a concrete image, addressing the question, What sort of people are we to be? The law was both gift and goal.

Jesus and Reciprocity: Power Gone Awry or Mercy?

In spite of the continued rejection of the divinely instigated and empowered vocation to reflect God's own character, that vocation has remained remarkably consistent. In the eighth century B.C.E., the prophet Amos actually accused Israel of looking too much like Egypt, so far had they departed from their vocation as a community. Yet God continued to lay before His people the same opportunity for relationship. According to the New Testament Gospels, the message of Jesus did not introduce anything markedly new in this regard; he was very much a traditionalist, repeating the message of the prophets, adopting a style of ethical teaching reminiscent of the already widespread wisdom tradition,[16] embracing the call to be God's covenant community. He also laid before them a vision of life together very much like that we have already encountered. In the example we will examine, the language has changed to reflect a different setting, now in the Rome-dominated world of ancient Palestine, but the message echoes the spirit of God's initial hope in creation.

In the midst of what is often called the Sermon on the Plain, Jesus says,

> But I say to you that listen, Love your enemies, do good to those who hate you, bless those who curse you, pray for those who

abuse you. If anyone strikes you on the cheek, offer the other also; and from anyone who takes away your coat do not withhold even your shirt. Give to everyone who begs from you; and if anyone takes away your goods, do not ask for them again. Do to others as you would have them do to you.

If you love those who love you, what credit is that to you? For even sinners love those who love them. If you do good to those who do good to you, what credit is that to you? For even sinners do the same. If you lend to those from whom you hope to receive, what credit is that to you? Even sinners lend to sinners, to receive as much again. But love your enemies, do good, and lend, expecting nothing in return. Your reward will be great, and you will be children of the Most High; for he is kind to the ungrateful and the wicked. Be merciful, just as your Father is merciful.[17]

As elsewhere in the Gospel of Luke, one finds here two approaches to life set over against one another.[18] On the one hand stands the agonistic, competitive form of life available to people throughout the ancient Mediterranean world. This was everyday life marked in part by the imbalance of patron-client relations, relationships of inequality characterized by claims of honor and status and by the exertion of power over others. Put simply, the potential patron had some commodity, whether tangible or not, required by a client. In exchange, the client provides appropriate expressions of honor and loyalty to the patron. The point is that, having received patronage, the client now existed in a state of obligation, of debt. The possibilities for exploitation and the exercise of controlling, coercive power are high.

Jesus sets himself and his message over against this way of life, contrasting the behaviors that characterize everyday life in his world with behaviors that grow out of service in the kingdom of God. The contrast is explicit in the structure of the passage we have cited above. First, he commands, "Love your enemies, do good to those who hate you," juxtaposing this statement with the question, "If you love those who love you, what credit is that to you?" Similarly, his charge, "Bless those who curse you, pray for those who abuse you. And if anyone strikes you on the cheek, offer the other one as well; likewise, if anyone takes your coat from you, do not hold back your shirt," is set over against his observation, "If you do good only to those who are good to you, what credit is that to you?" Finally, parallel to his assertion,

"Give to everyone who begs from you," stands his final question, "If you lend to those from whom you hope to receive in return, what good is that to you?" In each case, those whose goodness grows of the system of patronage—give to those who give to you, in order to build up a series of claims over others—are said to be no better than sinners. Here, as often in the Gospels, "sinners" are not simply "those who transgress the law," but, rather, "those whose behavior separates them from the group of reference"—i.e., "them," not "us." In this case, Jesus seems to be challenging his listeners not to act like outsiders, but like God's people. In doing so, he urges them to refuse the coercive, control-dominated system of relationships characteristic of the wider world.

Interestingly, it is not that Jesus disacknowledges how deeply ingrained in his world the patron-client system is. Instead, he not only recognizes that people of his culture understand that this is the way the world works, he actually capitalizes on this way of thinking. Thus, having juxtaposed two ways of relating to people in the world, he goes on to suggest why his audience should adopt this new set of behaviors: "Your reward will be great, and you will be children of the Most High." Jesus is actually working from *within* the model of benefaction here. He says, in effect: Give freely to one another, without expectation of return; relate to others with love and provide for their needs, without keeping a record of their obligation to you; for God will take up their cause, and He will pay you what is due; expect goodness from God, but do not hold over the head of your neighbors your claim on them.

This is not the end of the story, however. Jesus is trying to take the center of gravity for life away from the deeply rooted social systems of his day and to do so he is willing to use those systems while turning them on their head. At the same time, he is concerned to communicate a more fundamental motivation for gracious behavior: "God is kind to the ungrateful and the wicked. Be merciful, just as your Father is merciful." In other words, be like God in your actions. God does not withhold goodness from those who reject Him, from those who will not return His love. Neither should you. Let God's own character mold your character, your behavior.

As in the Deuteronomic material under review earlier, so here we find a direct line drawn from God's character to human behavior, from the Triune God to the human community. As in that context, so here, our making this connection depends on our gaining our resources and bearings for the caring life from the doxological life, the life of worship. Jesus' reference to "your Father" is an explicit reminder that we find our full humanity in relation to the God who made us and cares for us—a relationship modelled by Jesus above all else in his experience of God's Spirit, his life in the community of disciples, and his habits of corporate and personal prayer and worship.

This appeal to God's own character also underlies the radical quality of Jesus' remarkable admonition even to "love your enemies." Such an injunction flies in the face of the conventional wisdom by which we acknowledge the insensibility of failing to distinguish enemies from friends. Even if ancient sources counsel compassion for the enemy in need,[19] they provide only the most general context of moral attitude for Jesus' command. Jesus' words, "love your enemies," lack any commonly held ethical base and can only be understood as an admonition to conduct inspired by God's own graciousness. Now the *imago Dei* has become the *imitatio Dei*, the reflection of God's image is seen in behavior that imitates God.

Examples of the way in which ethical comportment is shaped fundamentally by God's character, particularly as God is experienced within the community of worship, could easily be multiplied. At this point, however, it may be more helpful to look in more depth at a central affirmation of classical Christian faith, the incarnation of God. What light might the presentation of this concept in the New Testament shed on our understanding of the caring life?

WORD MADE FLESH:
THE STORY OF INCARNATION AS A STORY OF CARE

The doctrine of the incarnation, that God became a human being in Jesus, occupies a position at the heart of Christian faith. Concern over how best to understand and articulate the mechanics of that transaction—How can Jesus be both human and divine, as the creeds affirm?—has unfortunately detracted from efforts within the Christian community to explore the meaning of the incarnation for day-to-day life. Indeed, studies of incarnational christology in the New Testament in recent years have approached the New Testament data from the standpoint of the speculative question, When and how did the doctrine of the incarnation originate?, without broaching the issue of the implications of Jesus' pre-existence and incarnation for wider issues of faith and life. Modern christology is not alone in its failure to recognize and exploit the ethical message of the incarnation, however.

John, the Fourth Evangelist, is the only Gospel writer who affirms unequivocally his belief in the pre-existence of Christ and incarnation of God. He asserts at the beginning of his Gospel that Jesus, the Word, "was God";[20] this testimony, taken together with the exalted picture of Jesus presented elsewhere in the Fourth Gospel, has led more than one New Testament scholar to argue for a docetic view of Christ in this book: Jesus was like a god striding upon the earth, not quite human.[21] Apparently, others in the first century read the Gospel of John in this way too, so that additional correspondence followed, affirming in no uncertain terms the humanity of Jesus and the this-worldly character of his ethic of love.[22] It appears that a devaluation of his status as a human had the consequence of a de-emphasis on the importance of a this-worldly morality. In fact, nothing could be further from the vision set forth by the Fourth Evangelist, as a close reading of the Gospel of John demonstrates.

The prologue to the Gospel of John (John 1:1–18) has intrigued its readers not least because of its fascination with a christological term for Jesus that never again appears in the Gospel. We are informed that Jesus is the "Word" or "Logos" in a way that underscores its paramount importance, only to have this language disappear from view as the Gospel narrative begins. A reading of John's language in its literary-cultural environment, with special reference to the Alexandrian Jew Philo, reveals that there is little about John's Logos that would be unfamiliar to those exposed to philosophical speculation about the "immanence of God." As at other times in history, so in the first century some people struggled with how to speak of God's nearness without compromising the reality of God's "holy otherness," his transcendence. One of the terms employed for "God as he draws near to us" was Logos, Word, and it is this language that Philo and John share. Conceptually, these two writers are very close, until one reaches what is for John the central affirmation: "The Word became flesh and lived among us."[23]

Clearly, John uses the Logos-concept as an entry point for his audience, bringing to mind previously known categories of speaking of God, in order to highlight the literal coming of God into the world in the form of God's own Son. In this way, John communicates that God's Son, Jesus, is God incarnate, God who has come into the world. After the prologue, one hears only of the Son of God, no longer of the Logos, but John's readers or auditors know that the Evangelist has begun defining the title "Son of God" with reference to the pre-existence and the entry into the world of the Logos.

The question remains, What is the purpose of this coming? Why has God entered the world? The subsequent narrative is told in such a way as to invite the reader to ask that very question. Repeatedly, we are told, the hour for which Jesus was sent is coming—or, that hour has not yet arrived. Thus, some Jerusalemites were angry with Jesus and wanted to arrest him, "but no one laid their hands on him, for his hour had not yet come." Again, while teaching in the temple, Jesus seemed to associate himself too intimately with God, an act for which he might have been disciplined, even put to death, "but no one arrested him, because his hour had not yet come." Still later, Jesus is troubled and wonders what to pray. "Shall I say, 'Father, save me from this hour'?" he asks. He answers his own question, "No, it is for this reason that I have come to this hour."[24] What is this hour? We are told that this "hour" is the hour of Jesus' glorification,[25] but what is this? How does the unfolding story provide signification for this "glorification," this "hour?"

Throughout the first half of the Fourth Gospel, the suspense has been building. John has staged the narrative in such a way as to build a crescendo of dramatic anticipation. What hour is coming? The answer comes, finally, in the famous scene of Jesus' last meal with his disciples, his washing the disciples' feet (John 13:1–17).

Footwashing was a mundane aspect of life in the first century. Walking on sandy paths with sandals created this simple necessity. When guests arrived, washing their feet was a sign of hospitality, so important in this society.[26]

This, however, was an agonistic, competitive society, one in which issues of status, of honor and shame, were integral to every social interaction. Washing the feet of another, then, was no simple enterprise, for one must always first struggle with the question, What is appropriate to a person of my social position? This was critical, since every social interaction became an opportunity for me to enhance my status, by making a claim for social honor that others around me recognized, or to be shamed. Who should wash whose feet? Jewish males should not wash someone else's feet, according to the Rabbis, not even the feet of a Jewish male. This was a task for Gentile slaves, or for women and children.

Given this social reality it is not surprising that, before the meal on the night narrated in John 13, no one offered to wash the feet of anyone else. By making no such offer, say, James and John did nothing extraordinary. They were simply making a claim to being status equals with the other disciples. So by the social conventions of their day, no one could blame them for their not having washed the feet of the others. The problem is that there was no one of lesser status present to handle this commonplace chore. To this matter we must return.

The introduction to this scene is pivotal for our understanding of the whole drama, so we will unpack it in stages.

After an initial chronological indicator, "it was just before the festival of the Passover", the first hint of the import of this story is provided: "Jesus knew that his hour had come to depart from this world and go to the Father." An initial answer to our earlier question is provided, for here we realize that the mysterious "hour" has to do with the completion of Jesus' journey from heaven to earth, and now from earth back to heaven. This, it would seem, is the "glorification" about which we read earlier. We must not think of this glorification in simple spatial terms, however; instead, we may continue to ask, In what consists Jesus' glorification? Or, more straightforwardly, What is the purpose of this journey, this coming into the world?

Onto this heavily laden issue of interpretation and significance around which the Gospel of John turns we may lay another one. John goes on to introduce the pending scene in a second way: "Having loved his own who were in the world, he now showed them the full extent of his love." That is, in the scene about to be narrated, John tells us, Jesus' love comes to full expression, it reaches its intended goal.[27]

Adding further significance to the coming story is a third introductory notation: "The devil had already put it in the heart of Judas son of Simon Iscariot to betray Jesus." Now we see that the coming events are the arena of cosmic assault, that the scene about to unfold is of eschatological significance.

How, then, will Jesus fulfill his mission? How will he complete his love? How will he engage in cosmic assault?

What can Jesus do that will carry this theological weight? What might he do that will have such extraordinary significance? John continues the story:

> During supper, Jesus . . . arose from the meal, took off his robe, and tied a towel around himself. Then he poured water into a basin and began to wash the feet of his disciples. . . .

We may recall that the fact that the disciples had not already washed each other's feet reflected societal norms. They were status equals.

But this makes Jesus' behavior all the more striking. As the disciples and he admit, he is their "Teacher" and "Lord"—that is, he is not their status equal, but their better. They follow him. He teaches them. He is the last person in that room who should be taking up basin and towel, as Peter belatedly acknowledges when he says to Jesus, "You will never wash my feet."

But this is how Jesus fulfills his mission. This is how he engages in cosmic battle. This is how he demonstrates to his community of followers the full extent of his care. This is how he receives glory from God: He washes the feet of those in his charge. He refuses to claim the benefits of higher status and openhandedly serves those below him on any scale of ranking. In doing so, he passes judgment on those attitudes, those communities, those systems that support human reluctance to embrace caring service, which instead honor stories of escape from positions of giving service to positions of being served. Jesus redefines the basis of status around living a life oriented toward others, and he provides a fresh image of the exercise of power as freedom to serve those previously defined as one's servants. He confirms by his behavior what we have repeatedly seen: It is the nature of God not to cling tightly to honor or status or rights, but to set these aside in order to care for those of lesser honor, lesser status, fewer rights. This is God's nature, and, by extension, the human vocation.

The words of Jesus at the close of this scene underscore this vision of the caring life:

> Do you know what I have done to you? You call me Teacher and Lord—and it is as you say, for I am these things. Therefore, if I, the Lord and Teacher, have washed your feet, you ought also to wash one another's feet.

In these words, Jesus underscores that the significance of this scene does not fall on the act of foot washing, as though this were the behavior his disciples lacked. Nor does he recommend that the subsequent church adopt (or recover) foot washing as a community-defining practice.[28] Rather, Jesus uses foot washing as an object lesson against seeking honor, claiming status, holding on to one's own rights. As Paul will later write, "Let the same mind be in you that was in Christ Jesus, who, though he was in the form of God, did not consider equality with God as something to be clutched, but emptied himself, taking the form of a slave. . . ."[29]

CONCLUSION

In an essay of this brevity, it has not been possible to develop fully a theological and biblical perspective on care, nor address with much specificity what attitudes and behaviors might qualify as "caring." The lack of greater attention to this latter issue, however, is less due to its magnitude than to the reality that "caring" can hardly be defined in the abstract. Just as we know the character of God only in the concreteness of our lives, especially within the community of God's people, so we recognize the threads and hues of human reflection of God's character only in the fabric of social life in the everyday world.

At the same time, we have insisted that any vision of fully human interaction must take as its point of departure the nature of God, and this precisely because it is in reflecting the divine nature that full humanity is experienced. This reality underscores the importance of attitudes and practices grounded in covenant love within the human family. It also speaks a strong word of judgment against social interaction, even that parading under the guise of "care," which is guided by status-based competition, rights-based individualistic claims, and other forms of coercive power. Affirmed are manifestations of disinterested care and practices that free others to lives wherein the promise of each is enabled and our common human vocation is furthered. The rootedness of the human vocation in the creation of humanity in the divine image also has as its corollaries (1) the significance of the doxological life as the requisite foundation for the caring life, and (2) the friendships and practices of the redeemed community as the context for its comportment. "Care" is God's gift to human beings, and within this gift is embodied both the call and capacity to be the community of care.

NOTES

Abbreviations:
> BTS   Biblisch Theologische Studien
> NRSV   New Revised Standard Version
> OBT   Overtures to Biblical Theology
> SNTSMS   Society for New Testament Studies Monograph Series
> WBC   Word Biblical Commentary

1. Luke 22:25–26. Unless otherwise noted, translations of biblical materials are my own.

2. See Suzanne Gordon, "A National Care Agenda," *The Atlantic* (January, 1991).

3. See, e.g., 1 Peter 2:21–25. Throughout this letter, the author appeals to Christian believers experiencing pervasive and painful social marginalization to (1) place their suffering in the interpretive context of Jesus' innocent suffering (cf. 4:12–13) and (2) maintain faithfulness in the world.

4. Didache 11:4–5, 9 (my translation). It may be that concerns of this nature have motivated the phraseology of Matthew 10:11.

5. Revelation 1:4, 8.

6. Genesis 1:26–27. Note in particular how Genesis 1 devotes attention to the narration of those aspects of God's creative activity that are of special help to human beings and the degree to which the narrative pace slows in Genesis 1:26–30.

7. Cf. William Hordern, "Man, Doctrine of," in *A Dictionary of Christian Theology*, ed. Alan Richardson, (London: SCM, 1969), 202–205.

8. Karl Barth, *Church Dogmatics*, vol. 3: *The Doctrine of Creation*, pt. 1 (Edinburgh: T. & T. Clark, 1958), 176–213.

9. Barth, *Church Dogmatics*, 3.1: 184–185.

10. This is not to suggest that the original narrator intended a Trinitarian reading of these first person plural pronouns, however; see the discussion in Gordon J. Wenham, *Genesis 1-15*, WBC 1 (Waco, TX: Word, 1987), 27–28.

11. Walter Brueggemann, *Genesis*, Interpretation (Atlanta: John Knox, 1982), 32.

12. On the meaning of "covenant love" (Hebrew: ‏ד ס ח‎), see the reappraisal in Francis I. Andersen, "Yahweh, the Kind and Sensitive God," in *God Who Is Rich in Mercy: Essays Presented to Dr. D.B. Knox*, ed. Peter T. O'Brien and David G. Peterson (Homebush West, New South Wales: Lancer/Anzea, 1986), 41–88; H. J. Zobel, "‏ד ס ח‎," in *Theological Dictionary of the Old Testament*, vol. 5, ed. G. Johannes Botterweck and Helmer Ringgren (Grand Rapids, MI: Wm. B. Eerdmans, 1986) 44–64.

13. See Norbert F. Lohfink, S.J., *Option for the Poor: The Basic Principle of Liberation Theology in the Life of the Bible* (Berkeley, CA: BIBAL, 1987).

14. Deuteronomy 24:19–22 NRSV.

15. Deuteronomy 6:4–5.

16. This is not to say that Jesus was not in his own way innovative in his ethics, but only to recognize that he worked very much within the framework of God's purposeful activity as presented in the Hebrew Scriptures. Cf. A.E. Harvey, *Strenuous Commands: The Ethic of Jesus* (London: SCM; Philadelphia: Trinity, 1990).

17. Luke 6:27–36 NRSV.

18. See further, Halvor Moxnes, *The Economy of the Kingdom: Social Conflict and Economic Relations in Luke's Gospel*, OBT (Philadelphia: Fortress, 1988).

19. Cf. John Piper, *Love Your Enemies: Jesus' Command in the Synoptic Gospels and the Early Christian Parenesis*, SNTSMS 38 (Cambridge: Cambridge University, 1979), ch. 2.

20. John 1:1.

21. See now, however, Marianne Meye Thompson, *The Humanity of Jesus in the Fourth Gospel* (Philadelphia: Fortress, 1988).

22. See 1 John.

23. John 1:14.

24. John 7:30; 8:20; 12:27; cf. 2:4; 4:21, 23; 5:25, 28; 12:23; 17:1.

25. John 12:23.

26. See Luke 7:36–50 (44).

27. The translation adopted by the NRSV, "he loved them to the end," does not do justice to the theological weight of the Greek phrase employed here (εἰς τέλος).   Jesus did not only "love his disciples up to the last moment of his life," but in this story expressed his love in a complete way. Cf. Reinier Schippers, "τέλος," in *New International Dictionary of New Testament Theology*, vol. 2, ed. Colin Brown (Grand Rapids, MI: Zondervan, 1976), 59–66.

28. Cf. Udo Schnelle, *Neutestamentliche Anthropologie: Jesus — Paulus — Johannes*, BTS 18 (Neukirchen-Vluyn: Neukirchener, 1991), 134–139, who discusses the connection between incarnation, footwashing, and the cross.

29. Philippians 2:5–6.

Listening with Care

MORRIS A. MAGNAN

Yes, Mrs. Clark and her family would make the perfect case for my public health nursing class, the last course I had to take to earn my Bachelor's Degree in Nursing. Even though Mrs. Clark had ended our first meeting almost before it began, I'd stood firm. She knew I'd be back. Later at home with reference and writer's manual, dictionary, a lecture on the history of black American families, and hot chocolate close at hand, my process paper began to take shape. In fact, I could smell the fragrance of a forthcoming "A". The nursing diagnoses flowed like honey, the interventions were clearly within my capabilities, and the outcomes fell into measurable, behavioral terms.

Frankly, after 12 years in nursing, with what I describe as a "rich" clinical background in critical care, I welcomed the change of pace in public health. It piqued my interest just at a time when critical care seemed little more than an endless round of shadow boxing with interns and residents.

Crossing the railroad tracks jarred me out of my reverie. After two more blocks, the large two-story house loomed before me, looking more ominous than I'd remembered. The broken dormer windows seemed to peer through the rain at my approaching car.

I made my way to Mrs. Clark's house, knowing that the tough-minded little old lady inside was not about to be manipulated, cajoled, pressured, or reasoned into anything some white boy from the easy side of the tracks had to say. I decided to keep it simple: just R and R—ritual and relationship.

A functionally blind, 76-year-old insulin-dependent diabetic with congestive heart failure, Mrs. Clark had been bedridden for seven years.

A shorter version of this exemplar was first published in the American Journal of Nursing February 1989, pp. 219–221 (Vol. 89 (2)219–221).

Her primary caregiver was an 11-year-old granddaughter who lived with her, prepared her meals, injected her with insulin every morning, and emptied the slop bucket brimming with the contents of her bedpan. For all her efforts, the child was rewarded only with Mrs. Clark's venomous tongue, the back of her hand, and her seemingly unpredictable wrath.

The family had been referred to the local Visiting Nurses' Association as a follow-up referral from Social Services when it was noted that the granddaughter was frequently absent from school because she had to stay home to care for her sick grandmother.

The house's condition was deplorable—no heat, no electricity, no hot water, no running water in the toilet. Accumulated furniture, clothing, newspapers, and Mrs. Clark's bed had reduced the living room space to two small pathways. Any distinction between trash and treasure was known only to Mrs. Clark. Mice and cockroaches showed no respect, trespassing at will over everything in the room.

And so we began. Mrs. Clark had agreed to let me in three times a week for 30 minutes to check her vital signs and measure her ankles. Collecting my assessment data took five minutes at most. Then I'd settle onto a pile of newspapers to listen to my "case study".

"Well, ain't no call in you just sittin'. Might just as well get on outta here," she jeered.

"Yes, ma'am. I'll be leaving in 25 minutes, just as we agreed," I'd counter. Two weeks later she was still trying to shoo me away.

"Well, if you're going to sit there you might just as well read something. You do know how to read don't you?"

"Yes," I answered, hoping I was reading the cues properly.

"If you were a Christian, you might try reading the Bible. You might learn something from it," she quipped.

I had not failed to notice the Bible beside her bed and without asking picked it up. "Personally, I like John's Gospel, but I see someone's marked a place in Proverbs," I said.

As I began to read she interrupted with, "That reminds me of when I first came here from Alabama back in '42 . . ." She went on to tell me about running away with her children to escape an alcoholic husband. She lived in a shelter and worked as a maid until she saved enough money to rent a house. Getting up early, she made home-cooked Southern style breakfasts for the local factory workers before going to her regular job. After two or three years she had saved enough money to start her own restaurant and bought the house she now lived in. From there she went on to buy six more rental homes in her neighborhood which she still owned and rented to the grandchildren she had raised. I marveled at her achievements and commented on how much courage it must have taken for a woman, especially a Black woman, to make it alone in the 40's, raise two families and run a business.

Mrs. Clark's sister met me at the door on my next visit. It was bath day, but Mrs. Clark refused to be bathed or eat her lunch.

"She's funny that way. Moody, you know. Can't nobody stand to be around her."

Sure enough, Mrs. Clark cursed at me and refused to let me check her blood pressure. She smacked my hand as I touched her cheek, but the cold, clammy skin I felt confirmed my suspicions. She was having an insulin reaction.

Once I explained the problem to Mrs. Clark's sister, she pitched in. We concocted a mixture of cream of wheat and plenty of sugar. Then started the funniest test of wills I had ever witnessed. Mrs. C. shaking her head, stubbornly refused to eat while she cursed her sister. Sister stood her ground unflinchingly. Poised patiently over her target, she smothered one profanity after another with heaping spoonfuls of cream of wheat. "Bull's eye," I shouted encouragingly from my stack of newspapers. "Thank you, Jesus," echoed Mrs. Clark's sister. Thus we proceeded in our unorthodox canticle to sweeten Mrs. Clark's blood sugar and hopefully her disposition.

Gradually, Mrs. Clark came around. Surprisingly, she apologized. Predictably, she refused to talk about going to the hospital or seeing a doctor. Mrs. Clark's sister agreed to stay with her to make sure she ate dinner and promised to come again the next day at noon to feed her lunch and talk to me.

The next day, the three of us sorted through Mrs. Clark's symptoms. After taking insulin for 20 years, Mrs. Clark was surprised to hear that feeling "woozy, jittery, mean and cold all over" was her way of manifesting hypoglycemia. All along she'd thought she was possessed by a demon.

No doubt the time was right for some dietary teaching, but instead I began some dietary learning. I started making extra visits to make sure the granddaughter was measuring the insulin correctly. We planned ways to stimulate Mrs. Clark's appetite; in fact, Mrs. Clark enjoyed dreaming about foods she wished she could eat. Mouth-watering wishing yielded one incredible exchange list of wetbread and grits, honey and corn muffins, buttermilk and kneebones, fried chicken and greens.

Soon our meetings took on a different flavor—that of victuals and vengeance. Mrs. Clark would uncover an array of home-cooked foods and finish them off with lots of lip-smacking relish. From my newspaper perch, I'd sweat it out, watching her put away one dish after another.

"Well now, Mr. Nurse, tell me more about that exchange list of yours."

That was my cue to sort the homemade masterpieces into food groups and estimate calories. How would I know how many calories are in a kneebone? Invariably, I'd fail.

"Well, maybe next time you'll know," she'd chide, the sweet taste of victory gleaming in her eyes.

We started having company regularly for lunch. Sharing a country background, Mrs. Clark and I traded stories, such as toe-testing the weight-bearing load of cow pies, much to the horror and delight of the granddaughters. And we'd fantasize about walking barefoot in spring grass until our feet turned green. Occasionally, I sat silent as Mrs. Clark cried with her granddaughters thinking about the past when her house was the cleanest one on the block, when she could work all day in her restaurant, walk the two miles home and still have enough energy to scrub her kitchen floor. "But now," she wept, "my house is falling down around me. And me stuck in this bed!"

Several days passed before the mystery of the home-cooked lunches was revealed to me.

"Gran'mama, I cooked everything just the way you said," the young woman shouted over her shoulder as she backed into the room struggling to catch the storm door in the wind.

"You're late!" The old woman's chilled voice froze the girl in her tracks. "Well, bring it over her," she commanded. Hesitantly, the young woman set her parcel down and eased her way back to the door.

"You can leave when I say you can leave. Sit down!" she ordered. Folding under the tension, the young woman sank down beside me on the newspapers. Together we sat in silence as Mrs. Clark ate her lunch. I guessed the young woman to be a granddaughter.

"Yolanda," snapped the old woman. "Come here where I can see you." Frightened, the young woman inched her way toward the unpredictable old lady. As she came within striking range the old woman shot out a hand grabbing the girl firmly by the wrist. Holding her fast, she pulled the struggling girl down to her and ever so softly kissed her on the cheek. "You done good baby. You done real good," she whispered. Surprised and confused, Yolanda left.

Before excusing me for the day, Mrs. Clark explained how she had managed to arrange her own "Meals on Wheels" by phoning her recipes to her granddaughters. I was never sure whether she persuaded them or terrorized them into cooperating, but the meals kept coming and so did the granddaughters.

I still hadn't quite understood why Mrs. Clark couldn't walk until one day a granddaughter whispered a family secret.

"Gran'mama was laying on her daybed when the police came to tell us my brother had been killed. That was seven years ago, and she hasn't been out of that bed since." So that was it.

Wrestling with this information for several days, I concluded that I could not be a part of the silent conspiracy.

"Tell me about your grandson," I ventured one day. She searched the stillness of the room.

"It doesn't matter who told me, Mrs. Clark, I know. I also know you loved him very much and I want to hear you talk about how much you loved him." I stayed long over my allotted time that day. I lost track of the comings and goings of the granddaughters, but somehow the message got out and the food began to arrive. A small crowd huddled around Mrs. Clark rocking her and hugging her and encouraging her to cry it all out. The words of love and encouragement drew the others into their own experience of grief and healing. As they paired-off to the comfort of each other's arms, I reminisced about some of my own losses. In time the family remembered . . . the wave in his hair, the tone of his skin, his smile, his walk, his ways. Then one, then another told stories of their most cherished memories of Joshua.

Mrs. Clark began the weight-bearing exercises on my next visit. Confinement had certainly taken its toll on Mrs. Clark's legs, and I suspected some peripheral neuropathy from her diabetes had made matters worse. "Put your arms around me like you know me real well," I encouraged. After two weeks of exercise, Mrs. Clark could get from bed to chair with help and take lunch out of bed. She agreed to at-home physical therapy for gait training.

My instructor accompanied me on my last visit. The house was a hubbub of activity. Mrs. Clark's eldest son had moved in and was whitewashing the dining room. The granddaughters had cleared away many a "treasure" and were fixing up a downstairs bedroom for Gran'mama. Amidst all this activity, I described my taking vital-signs, measuring ankles, transferring Mrs. Clark to a chair and then just sitting through lunch and listening. It didn't sound like much, especially since my clinical evaluation hinged on this last visit alone.

"So you came anyway," Mrs. Clark snapped. "Last day, I thought you might not come." Mrs. Clark was in wicked form.

"I want to check your blood pressure, Mrs. Clark," I stammered.

"Go on then, do what you have to," Mrs. Clark griped.

I kept my back to my instructor, hoping she wouldn't see my embarrassment, and quickly went through my routine.

"Can I help you into your chair?" I offered.

"Don't need your help. You ain't comin' back no more anyway. Just hand me my walker."

In amazement, I watched Mrs. Clark pull herself up with the walker, shuffle through the most magnificent pivot I'd ever seen, and sit down in her chair.

Ritual and relationship indeed.

Philosophical Reflections on Caring Practices

CHARLES TAYLOR

The contributors to this book approach the subject of caring from their particular experiences and particular areas of expertise, some in a theoretical fashion and others in a testimonial fashion. My own discipline is philosophy. I will attempt to address what is involved in fighting for, struggling for, and overcoming the crisis of care and making it more possible for people to care again and carry out caring within the caring professions. In so doing, I will bring into the discussion what philosophers and philosophical thought have to contribute to this struggle.

In an early chapter Robert Bellah wrote about the kind of society we live in, the obstacles this society creates to taking caring seriously, and the reasons why caring seems to be marginalized in our society today. The problem is complicated and exists on many levels. Bellah referred to the work of Jurgen Habermas who identifies two kinds of institutions in our society that operate in impersonal ways and, in a way, make decisions for us or remove from our shoulders responsibility for certain decisions. Though we sometimes view this situation negatively, we also play along with it because it has positive benefits for us.

In order to be the kind of human beings we want to be we have to understand how these mechanisms operate, what they do to us, and what we have to do back to them. The two mechanisms are the market and what Habermas sometimes calls the state, though it is more than that. I call the second mechanism "bureaucratic ways of proceeding" or "ways of proceeding by bureaucratic rules." These are rules that are laid down, become rigid, and must be followed. For brevity's sake, I will refer to the two mechanisms as "market" and "bureaucracy." Habermas claims they are powerful steering mechanisms because they lift the burden of decision off us. We can see this clearly in the case of the market when we look at the recently collapsing communist societies.

In a sense, the dream of Marxism (or of Leninist and Stalinist variants of it) was to go beyond the market, to take back those decisions about what is to be produced and how that is to be allocated and distributed. The dream was to take those decisions back from the market and make them collectively through some kind of planning authority of the state. We know the disaster brought about by attempting to do that in a total way. That is what we are seeing today. So we learn that markets are in some way essential to modern societies. Modern industrialist societies require efficacy, and this necessitates the market.

However, I must say that the present mindless self-congratulation of Western society in the face of the collapse of communist societies misses the point. The sort of Thatcher-Reagan idea that everything can be done by markets makes as little sense as the Leninist belief that nothing should be done by markets. It is evident that the challenge is to find ways to combine the market and the bureaucracy.

Those who favor the market stress the necessity of the market for efficacy and also for a negative kind of freedom that enables each individual to move around and make arrangements for his or her life. This freedom is not total by any means. It is very restricted within a market-based regime, but there is a greater degree of this kind of freedom within such a regime than in a regime in which everything is planned from the center. Markets must play a role within societies because they contribute efficacy and negative freedom.

In the cases of market rule and bureaucratic rule one sees that decisions are taken away from individual people. Certain features of the overall patterns of distribution and production result from an interplay of decisions and are, in a sense, in their aggregate form decided by nobody. Decisions are taken away from people, but they are not given to other people. They are left to the play of impersonal forces.

Within bureaucratic rule certain decisions are taken away from individuals who are required to follow sets of rules. The requirement that rules be followed precludes the possibility of scrapping the rules, finding alternative ways of making decisions, or taking a shortcut to a decision. As with market rule, the decisions are taken away from individuals and not given to any other particular person. The decisions repose in some impersonal institution. This process is forced, in part, by the demands of efficacy, although some applications of bureaucracy produce inefficacy. Large-scale operations requiring large-scale coordination make decision making impossible without some degree of set rules. Bureaucracy becomes important to keep everything from grinding to a halt. In addition to the demand for efficacy, bureaucracy is seen to be necessitated by the demand for fairness. People see bureaucracy as necessary to make sure that people's rights are not trampled on, that everyone is able to be heard, and that everyone's rights are taken into account.

Behind these powerful steering mechanisms within our society—the market and bureaucracy—are our deep commitments to particular goals and ideals, such as efficacy, fairness, individual freedom, and individual rights. Efficacy, fairness, freedom, and rights form an ethos that helps drive the steering mechanisms. They keep us in line, and it is our commitment to these goals and ideals that spreads outward from our civilization and has made it impossible for the East to deny the market. However gloomy this view, it is my belief that the Eastern states (the Soviet Union, the other Eastern European states, and, eventually, China) were brought down more by their poor economic performance than by their human rights records. The Soviet Union's poor economic performance forced Gorbachev into *perestroika* as people lost faith in the state as an engine of progress. Subsequent to that loss of faith, the state's dismal human rights record and systematic mendacity weighed heavily on the people. The state's failure to meet the economic need for growth is what was decisive in the demise of the Soviet Union.

We, too, in the West hold the goals and ideals of efficacy, fairness, freedom, and rights. It would be hard for most of us to live in a society without the steering mechanisms of the market and bureaucracy. In making those goals and ideals our whole horizon, a society is created that accentuates individual freedom and procedural liberalism and is flawed in ways illustrated by other contributors to this book. Procedural liberalism does not concern itself with substantive goals in people's lives, but rather acts as a traffic director coordinating resources that enable people to work toward their own life goals. In such a society efficacy is a goal everyone can agree on, because if we can increase the powers of the society as a whole, we can increase what we can distribute to all individuals as the means to carry out their own life plans.

One of the reasons for our commitment to growth in Western societies is that issues of fairness and distribution become easier to resolve if we have regular increments of growth. It is easier to take from the wealthy and give to the less well-off if what one takes from the wealthy comes from their increase in wealth. Now that we are in an economic climate of relative recession, taking from the wealthy is more difficult and people are less willing to agree to taxes for redistributive purposes.

In a society like our own, which is driven by efficacy, fairness, rights, and freedom, there is a push toward procedural liberalism. These four pressures are institutional. In addition to the institutional pressures, there are intellectual pressures that are generated out of this form of society and help to shape it. There are two of these intellectual pressures worth elaborating here; they operate together and can be examined separately. One of these intellectual pressures is the philosophy of the individual that understands social relations and larger social entities as put together by the choices and actions of individuals. This deeply entrenched philosophical vision holds individual freedom—negative freedom—as the highest value.

Another similarly deeply entrenched intellectual habit or outlook characteristic of our kind of society is that of understanding human life in terms of a single principle of explanation. Single principle explanations work against complex, multi-faceted understandings of human life, but they benefit from association with the tremendous prestige of natural science explanations that, to outsiders of science, seem to reduce complex phenomena to single principles and laws. We attempt to reproduce this scientific elegance in our thinking about human lives through the theory of procedural liberalism, which currently dominates political philosophy in the English-speaking world and is supported by very considerable thinkers, like John Rawls.

The theory of procedural liberalism emanates from our kind of society. It enshrines the values of efficacy, fairness, rights, and freedom. It has immense intellectual prestige because it seems to derive all ethical and political decisions from a single principle. The power of procedural liberalism is enormous for it carries the force of our major institutions, the force of our major moral ideals, and the force of our scientific intellectual ideals. It is a powerful adversary, but we who are concerned with the crisis of care within our society know it must be fought. We also know that the feet of procedural liberalism are made of clay. The ideals and institutions that compose it are not sufficient, even on their own terms, for human life in our society.

For instance, the market in Western society would not survive were it not enframed with nonmarket entities. Market relations need some ethic of honesty built into the people who participate in them. For markets to operate, the people participating in them must adhere to ethics of keeping one's word and obeying one's contracts. Markets, if they are going to be productive, require a culture of productive entrepreneurship, not criminal entrepreneurship, or the entrepreneurship of takeovers and asset stripping, or capital flight to foreign countries.

The market would not produce what people want if it were not situated within a culture with ethical institutions and commitments that are not determined by the market. The market does not operate on its own. It is enframed by the nonmarket bounds of the society that consist of aspects of the society (commitments, ideals, goals, values, institutions) that are thought to be of supreme importance—more important than the market itself. Such enframing has to happen on the institutional level and on the level of the laws of the society.

Enframing can operate through actual laws and provisions of the society by taking certain things (e.g., health care) out of the market or by restricting how markets operate. This enframing must be compatible with the people's understanding of human life and what is important for that. If within the society people understand themselves as individuals relating to and competing with other individuals, then it will not work to remove something like health care from the market; that is, people will not relate to that institution with the appropriate spirit. An example of a case like this is what happened to the public health service in Leninist societies.

A perverse result of Leninism was that by denying the market everywhere, it destroyed any ethos of limitation of the market. Consequently, in many Leninist societies the public health service, which was theoretically out of the market, was in actual fact the scene of such terrible corruption that hospital patients were unable to get sheets or medical attention without tipping the porters and other hospital workers. In this kind of situation, the market will creep back in even though the public health service has been legally removed from the market. The laws removing the public health service from the market were inadequate because there was not an ethos supporting it. The people acted out of a sense of despair and cynicism about public institutions and scrambled to serve their own interests. The public health service needed to be enframed by laws and by an understanding of health service for the public that would protect it from market forces. We must struggle to enframe certain institutions legally, and we must struggle on the level of the hearts and minds that bear our society's understandings of human life. We need to struggle and win on both levels.

Staying with the example of health care, the British system and my own Canadian system are characterized by a public health care service that delivers the greater part of health care without cost to the person in need because the cost is assumed by all the citizens of the country. Though far from perfect, this system seems to me to be greatly superior to a system that does not bring the whole society into the regimen. It is very difficult to enframe market relations if the whole society is not included. If you try to do so by having the larger, more successful and affluent part of the society engaging in market relations for health care and then ask that they help the people that cannot purchase health care, then you are asking the majority of citizens to subscribe to the proposition of charity. The majority are to transfer their goods to people they do not know. This is an extremely abstract proposition to ask people to assume.

One might think that people ought to rise to the occasion of charity and that the middle class and the affluent two-thirds of the society ought to be ready to vote the taxes necessary to give adequate care to all, but it does not usually work that way in any society, and the United States is not exceptional in this failure of charity. I do not know any other Western country where the affluent two-thirds of the society would vote the taxes necessary to give adequate care to all citizens. The reason that some other Western countries do have a better health care system is that the health care system was not put there as a measure whereby the affluent two-thirds are doing their duty and helping the less well-off. The system was put there with the understanding that this is a system for the common benefit of everyone. Then, once the system is in place, it is irremovable. If the Canadian government tried to remove our national health care system, it would incite a political revolution among the middle class.

There is an important general lesson for us in the politics of bringing about care, and that is a lesson in creating democratic majorities. When you have a system of impersonal mechanisms, like those of the market, that is producing some bad consequences for a small group of people, it is a mistake to focus on those consequences in such a way that the interests of a minority of people become pitted against the general welfare. The majority of people are going to think to themselves, "Well, the market works pretty well for most of us. Why should we go out of our way to destroy this system in order to do our duty by this minority? They can ask something of us, but not too much." That kind of framing of the issue will create a climate of opinion in which most people feel that unreasonable demands are being made on them.

To illustrate the better approach of creating democratic majorities, let us now examine an example from the field of ecological policy. Great leaps forward have been taken within this domain during the last twenty years. Twenty years ago there was a situation in which a number of cases involved small groups of people from particular localities fighting in defense of particular wilderness areas. The fights were defined as these local people wanting to have their habitats kept intact. It was framed as an issue of these people's aesthetico-ecological interests against the GNP or the prosperity of the whole country in general. It looked unreasonable that these people's preferences should take precedence over and trump the general interest in the growth of the country.

What happened to transform this situation in many cases was the general understanding of the population as a whole that the wilderness areas were important and worth preserving for the sake of all the citizens, not just for certain people who lived near them. In one case, the aboriginal people in the Queen Charlotte Islands off the coast of British Columbia were fighting to keep the islands from being utterly savaged by logging companies. Instead of operating as a small group of preservationists, they became the kernel of a large coalition that spanned the country. The general interest of the country was redefined in such a way that the preservation of the islands did not compete with the general interest, but, rather, served it. With this transformation of people's understanding of the general interest, suddenly we stopped losing some of these ecological preservation battles, and started winning them.

This sort of transformation is what is required in the field of care. If we define it as simply in the interest of the least advantaged in the society for the society to care more, then we must call on the advantaged majority to care more and to care more in an impersonal way because they do not know those for whom they are called to care. We would tell the advantaged people to care more in this impersonal way, to pay out the money, raise the taxes, vote appropriately, and so on. Such a system will not make the kind of headway we would see if the issue of care were redefined in terms of the general interest of the country. We need to struggle to redefine the health care delivery system as making health care more humane for everyone. The institution of health care delivery needs to be taken out of the market and enframed so that it is seen as part of the general interest. Withdrawing it from the market alone is not sufficient; it is the enframing that will prevent the slow creep of the market back into health care.

On the level of the cultural struggle in which we are engaged for the hearts and minds of ourselves and our fellow citizens, we must redefine what human life is about. We must fight for a view of human life that does not derive from the single principle of disengaged reason and one that holds the values of efficacy, fairness, rights, and freedom exclusively. This cultural struggle must be faced across the whole society, but the battles are fought in particular localities, in a hospital, in a school, in a church. It is only when the battles are fought in the particular localities that the influence will spill out to the minds and hearts of others and be shaped by encounters with the broader consciousness of our society.

It is here where philosophy can help. The dominant philosophy of our time is procedural liberalism. People who want to go against the culture of procedural liberalism in their work as nurses or teachers or doctors often become discouraged in battling the dominant culture. They begin to wonder if there is something wrong with them for being so out of tune with the majority and for feeling such apparently unjustified feelings. Philosophy can serve the negative function of picking some holes in procedural liberalism and showing these discouraged people that this dominant philosophy does not really stand up to scrutiny.

Philosophy can serve this critical function, and it can offer alternatives. Of course, it is not only philosophy that can do this. Patricia Benner's article has been a magnificent work of articulation. In her work she helps nurses articulate their experience in language that really captures the experience for them. They have been living these experiences, but the language they have had for them from medicine and nursing has been inappropriate to describe what they live and know. The language of cost-effectiveness and of much professional training negates the experience these nurses have of caring and does not express what their own life is about and what is of value in it. The nurses have not always been able to counter this dominant language, but Dr. Benner's work of articulation enables them to do so. Through this work the narratives of some nurses who are able to do this articulation are passed from place to place so other nurses can take up the stories, see themselves in them, and create their own stories. This releases the tremendous energy of people's life experience, which suddenly can express itself properly because it has words for itself. Through this expression it affirms itself and passes on to others, empowering them to do the same. The articulation of life experience can change people's whole experience of their situation. This word that comes from experience is empowering.

Philosophy has to do with discovering empowering words and, in particular, with the dimension of articulating experience in narrative. There is, however, much work to be done along this line in moral philosophy. Interwoven into the view of political life that I have called procedural liberalism is the notion that within moral life the main issue is how one acts, whether rightly or wrongly. Within this view, therefore, moral philosophy is concerned primarily with discovering the criteria by which a person can discover the criteria for determining how to act rightly. This is related to the intellectual quest for a single principle of moral life from which all right action can be deduced.

Like the nurses or teachers whose experience of caring does not fit into the framework of cost-effectiveness and efficacy they have been handed, we all as moral agents live richer moral lives than what is described in official philosophy. These lives we live are richer because our sense of morality is not concerned only with how we act. How we act is also a matter of how we are. In a sense paradoxically, how we act is a matter of who we are. Just think of what we mean when we talk about caring: at the core of caring is a way of being among others in which you can care for others, can be sometimes moved by others in the kind of way that is movingly described in the narratives in this book. It is that being moved by the other person that cannot be programed. It cannot happen all the time, but what would caring look like in a world where we were not moved by others? What would motivate caring action? What would give power to caring?

There are other motivations besides being moved by the other that could empower caring action. People can have terribly strong

moral principles that they feel they must live up to, such as the impersonal demand to always give of themselves. People can also have
strong ego ideals dictating caring action, and these ego ideals would
cause them shame if they did not live up to them. There are people
who believe our moral fuel, so to speak, ought to be moral principle
or ego ideals. I, however, believe that the goads to moral action motivated by moral principle and ego ideals are guilt and shame. Guilt
and shame are inadequate motivators. They do not inspire people to
care in the same way as being moved by the other does, and they are
dangerous.

As Nietzsche and other great contenders of morality have
pointed out, a stance of benevolence and caring for others that is
fueled by guilt often is accompanied by deep contempt for and disin-
terest in the people being helped. The person caring for the other is
not doing so out of respect or concern for the other, but, rather, is striving to live up to a principle or ideal. Care that is carried out without a
sense of the real worth of the recipient is flawed in the most profound
way. Such care can produce a sense of belittlement and, so, be destructive of the person toward whom it is directed. In the end, the stance of
caring needs to be motivated, at least from time to time, by the understanding of the other person as a lovable and worthy human being.
Theresa Stephany's and Tom Boyce's narratives in this book are moving for me because they show people being touched by and moved to
care for others who they see as lovable. Theresa Stephany was able to
act as she did because she was moved by the husband and wife. Tom
Boyce came to see Blake through the eyes of his mother who found
her son beautiful. If we do not have moments like that, I believe, it is
impossible to carry on in the stance of care. In a movie about Mother
Teresa, she is asked how she can care for the sick, dying, afflicted people for whom she cares. She answers, "Well, you know, they are made
in the image of God." When I saw that I thought, "She really believes
that!" That is what struck me. In a sense, theoretically as a believing
Christian, I believe that, too. But Mother Teresa does not just hold that
belief; she experiences people in that way, as made in God's image.
She is not living only from principles and ideals. Her whole life experience stands behind her caring actions. To look at the issue of morality simply in terms of how one acts is to reduce it too much. It is what
one "acts out of" that can make all the difference to how one acts. The
truly important question is how one manages to see human beings as
worthy, as eliciting of love. No one but God can manage this way of

seeing and loving all the time, but we can all do it some of the time. Making this way of experiencing others as worthy ought to be a key question for moral philosophy.

There are various influences in our moral lives that can help us experience others as worthy. Seeing other people who care in this way helps us to do likewise. My seeing Mother Teresa in the film made a difference in my capacity to care for others and see them as worthy. Philosophers also have specific contributions to make to moral philosophy that can help us all realize that understanding why something or someone is good can empower one to love it more. This is what I am concerned with when I discuss moral sources. Though difficult to articulate, a moral source is something that when turned toward and articulated can empower one to act in a way prescribed by the full moral view.

All moralities draw on moral sources, though much contemporary moral philosophy is impoverished by its neglect of moral sources. The importance of moral sources is evident in theistic morality in which God is, in a sense, such a moral source. For Plato the idea of the good is such a moral source, and in turning toward it people become empowered to act according to the good. One might think that, since secular humanist moralities do not look toward God or the good, they do not contain moral sources. However, if you observe how these moralities work in people's lives and listen to the rhetoric they employ when they invoke these moralities, then it becomes clear that the moral source is still there, though it has been displaced. For instance, in secular humanist moralities the dignity of the free, disengaged, self-choosing person operates like a moral source. When those who hold these moral positions invoke this understanding of human dignity in a way that inspires them to act out of their morality, then they are operating on the basis of their moral sources. All people act based on moral sources, and philosophy can help articulate these sources. Some great philosophers have helped us in precisely this way. Plato articulated his own version of moral sources and made it possible for people to act in the way they thought they ought to act. This is how moral philosophy can empower moral action. Philosophy also can disempower. A philosophy that negates moral sources altogether and turns people away from them disempowers people to act morally. How does this action of philosophy in bringing out moral sources and empowering moral action relate to the political action, discussed earlier, of building majorities in our society that make caring more possible? This question brings us to the huge issue of the plurality of moral sources and how we deal with it. We live in a society in which some people believe in God and others do not; some people are Christians and others are not; and some people have one form of secular humanism, while others have another form. These moral sources are significantly different. When we want to bring people with differing moral sources into coalitions supporting agreed-upon political or social programs, we must take into account the different kinds of moral sources that are animating the people.

All of us have histories in our respective moral and spiritual views of considering everyone else's view erroneous. Christians used to think that other people just lacked the moral source necessary for morality. Even today I have people ask me if people who do not believe in God can be moral. Conversely, some unbelievers have been tempted to think that people who believe in God are twisted and incapable of any kind of correct moral view. These attitudes are absurd. We need to go beyond this view of the other as incapable of morality. The ecumenical challenge is to recognize that we must live with, work with, and be in relative commerce with people from these different positions. Going further, we need to learn to feel and appreciate the force of moral sources we do not share.

This does not mean reducing the differences in the other positions and deciding the other positions are really our own position dressed up differently, for example, a Christian reading the Buddhist scriptures and deciding their message is the same as that of the Christian scriptures. That is a form of ethnocentrism or spiritual-family-centrism—being centered on one's own spiritual family. The other form of this moral myopia is thinking that outside of one's own particular view no one else has a moral view or at least not one that is worth mentioning. What we need in place of this spiritual or moral self-centeredness is the capacity to sense the power of the other's view, recognizing that it is not one's own and probably never will be. Gaining this capacity is made difficult for Christians looking at secular humanists because, in our civilization, secular humanism has immured itself in the inadequate moral philosophy of procedural liberalism whereby it does not even recognize the presence of its own moral sources and how they empower secular humanists. This fact puts writers like myself in the ridiculous and presumptuous position of trying to articulate for these secular humanists what their own moral sources are. I am acutely uncomfortable playing this role, but there does not seem to me to be any other alternative.

In order to carry out a real act of understanding that will allow those of us who are not secular humanists to treat those who are with all the dignity they deserve, we, perhaps, need to make descriptions of what they are about that they themselves are not making and may not want to make. This is how we can approach the possibility of forming a coalition around a political or social program that consists of believers and nonbelievers. We can coexist only if we have this capacity to reach out and feel the force of one another's moral views, gain real respect for each other, and develop a comradeship that will serve the program. Taking this even further, we must understand with deep sympathy the moral views of our adversaries, that is, people totally within the purview of procedural liberalism.

This demand to understand sympathetically these adversaries is implicit in what I have argued so far. Also, such an understanding enables us to discover the sources of procedural liberalism's moral values and see that they are richer and more like what we want to address than many may realize. That is, if one examines why people hold negative freedom as an important value, one is led to the very rich sources in the Western tradition beneath modern views of people as self-determining beings who find their own identities. If one looks even more closely at what it is to discover who one is, one sees that that can only happen in relationship to others, and, when this is seen, the negative libertarian position that nullifies community begins to dissolve. It is no accident that this modern epoch in which we think in terms of self-determining freedom and people finding themselves is also the epoch in which people are profoundly concerned with the need for recognition and identity through recognition. These two aspects of the modern epoch are linked and did not arise in the same culture and civilization by accident. Only people who live within an extremely narrow libertarian philosophy do not see the links between them.

I have just illustrated how trying to understand the negative libertarians as sympathetically as possible will have the effect of shaking some of their dogmas. We should struggle for this kind of understanding. It would be blind and self-defeating to write off people who hold other philosophical positions. It is only when we strive to understand them at their best that we can discover that, at the roots of their beliefs, are some of the concerns that are of absolutely central importance to us as well.

The political struggle to form majorities around issues and programs connects with this cultural struggle for understanding through which are shaped our own views and other's views about what human life is. We carry on these struggles in the ways we practice, in the ways we articulate our human experience, and in the ways we organize our philosophy. These two struggles have to be closely related in order to achieve the shift toward greater and better caring.

Contributors

Mima Baird, Ph.D., is a clinical psychologist in private practice in Walnut Creek, California.

Robert N. Bellah, Ph.D., is Elliott Professor of Sociology at the University of California, Berkeley. His most recent books include the coauthored *Habits of the Heart* and *The Good Society*.

Patricia Benner, R.N., Ph.D., F.A.A.N., is Professor in the Department of Physiological Nursing at the University of California, San Francisco. Her books include From *Novice to Expert: Excellence and Power in Clinical Nursing Practice* and (with Judith Wrubel) *The Primacy of Caring: Stress and Coping in Health and Illness*.

W. Thomas Boyce, M.D., is a pediatrician, Professor in Residence, Department of Pediatrics, School of Medicine, and the Director of the Department of Behavioral and Developmental Pediatrics at the University of California, San Francisco.

Jaime Escalante is a teacher of mathematics at Hiram Johnson Junior High School in Sacramento, California. He is the subject of the film *Stand and Deliver*.

Douglass E. Fitch, M.Div., Ph.D., is the senior pastor of Downs Memorial United Methodist Church in Oakland, California.

Joel B. Green, M.Div., Ph.D., is Associate Professor of New Testament at the American Baptist Seminary of the West and Graduate Theological Union, Berkeley, California. His recent books include *The Theology of the Gospel of Luke, Dictionary of Jesus and the Gospels, and The Death of Jesus: Tradition and Interpretation in the Passion Narrative*.

Morris H. Magnan, R.N., B.S.N., is a clinical nurse preceptor in the surgical intermediate care unit at Harper Hospital in the Detroit Medical Center, Detroit, Michigan.

Harvey Peskin, Ph.D., is a clinical psychologist in private practice in Berkeley, California, and is on the teaching faculty at San Francisco State University.

Eugene H. Peterson, M.Div., D.H.L., is a Presbyterian pastor and Professor of Spiritual Theology at Regent College in Vancouver, British Columbia. He is the author of many books, including *A Long Obedience in the Same Direction* and *Working the Angles*.

Susan S. Phillips, Ph.D., is Dean and Professor of Sociology at New College Berkeley in Berkeley, California, and Assistant Clinical Professor, School of Nursing, University of California, San Francisco. She is currently writing a book on critical caring practices in nursing with Patricia Benner and Judith Wrubel.

Anna E. Richert, Ph.D., is Associate Professor of Education, Department of Education, Mills College in Oakland, California. Currently she holds a Spencer Fellowship awarded by National Academy of Education and serves on the advisory board for the National Center for Research on Teacher Learning.

Sandi Schaffer is a K-12 teacher on special assignment for the East Bay Conservation Corps in northern California.

Lynn M. Schimmel, M.S., N.P., is a women's health nurse practitioner at Women's Health Associates in Davis, California.

Theresa Stephany, R.N., M.S., is a staff nurse at the Hospice Unit, Kaiser Permanente Hospital, Hayward, California.

E. Dawn Swaby-Ellis, M.D., is a pediatrician and Professor of Pediatrics at Emory University School of Medicine in Atlanta, Georgia. She is the author of *Sanctity of Life*.

Charles Taylor, Ph.D., is Professor of Political Science and Philosophy at McGill University in Montreal, Quebec. His books include *Hegel, Sources of the Self,* and *The Ethics of Authenticity.*

David C. Thomasma, Ph.D., is the Fr. Michael I. English, S.J., Professor of Medical Ethics and Director of the Medical Humanities Program at the Stritch School of Medicine at Loyola University Medical Center, Chicago, Illinois. His books include *For the Patient's Own Good: The Restoration of Beneficence in Health Care* (with Edmund D. Pellegrino) and *Human Life in the Balance*.

William Visick, M.D., was an anesthesiologist in San Francisco, California, at Letterman Hospital (1972–1974), Mt. Zion Hospital, and Pacific Prebyterian Medical Center (1975–1989).